Bleeding Disorders and Dentistry

Branislav V. Bajkin
Editor

Bleeding Disorders and Dentistry

Springer

Editor
Branislav V. Bajkin
University of Novi Sad, Faculty of Medicine,
Dentistry Clinic of Vojvodina
Novi Sad, Serbia

ISBN 978-3-032-26712-2 ISBN 978-3-032-26713-9 (eBook)
https://doi.org/10.1007/978-3-032-26713-9

This Springer imprint is published by the registered company Springer Nature Switzerland AG
The registered company address is: Gewerbestrasse 11, 6330 Cham, Switzerland

Contents

Abbreviations

5-HT	5-Hydroxytryptamine (serotonin)
ADP	Adenosine diphosphate
AF	Antifibrinolytics
ALK-1	Activin receptor-like kinase 1
aPCC	Activated prothrombin complex concentrates
A-PRF	Advanced platelet rich fibrin
aPTT	Activated partial thromboplastin time
AT	Antithrombin (earlier antithrombin III)
ATP	Adenosine triphosphate
BOP	Bleeding on probing
BSS	Bernard Soulier syndrome
BT	Bleeding time
BU	Bethesda units
cAMP	Cyclic adenosine monophosphate
CBC	Complete blood count
CBCT	Cone beam computed tomography
CFCs	Clotting factor concentrates
CNS	Central nervous system
COX-1	Cyclooxigenase-1
COX-2 inhibitors	Cyclooxygenase-2 inhibitors
Da	Dalton
DAPT	Dual antiplatelet therapy
DDAVP	Desmopressin, 1-deamino-8-D-arginin vasopressin
DIC	Disseminated intravascular coagulation
DMFT	Decayed, missing, and filled teeth index
DOACs	Direct oral anticoagulants
DTIP	Drug-induced immune thrombocytopenia
DVT	Deep venous thrombosis
EACA	Epsilon aminocaproic acid
EDTA	Ethylene diamine tetraacetic acid
ELISA	Enzyme-linked immunoassay
FBC	Full blood count
FC	Flow cytometry
FFP	Fresh frozen plasma

FI	Coagulation factor I
FIX	Coagulation factor IX
FV	Coagulation factor V
FVIII	Coagulation factor VIII
FXI	Coagulation factor XI
FXIII	Coagulation factor XIII
GBI	Gingival bleeding index
GP	Glycoprotein
GT	Glanzmann thrombasthenia
GvHD	Graft-versus-host disease
HCCC	Hemophilia comprehensive care center
HHT	Hereditary hemorrhagic telangiectasia
HIT	Heparin-induced thrombocytopenia
HIV	Human immunodeficiency virus
HLA	Human leukocyte antigen
HMWK	High molecular weight kininogen
HPA	Human platelet antigen
HSP	Henoch-Scönlein purpura
HUS	Hemolytic uremic syndrome
IANB	Inferior alveolar nerve block
IgA	Immunoglobulin A
INR	International Normalized Ratio
I-PRF	Injectable platelet rich fibrin
ITI	Immune tolerance induction
ITP	Immune thrombocytopenic purpura
IU	International units
IVIgG	Intravenous immunoglobulin gamma
Liquid-PRF	Liquid platelet rich fibrin
LMWHs	Low molecular weight heparins
L-PRF	Leukocyte platelet-rich fibrin
LTA	Light transmission aggregometry
MELD	Model for End-Stage Liver Disease
NO	Nitric oxide
NSAIDs	Non-steroidal anti-inflammatory drugs
ONRC	Oxidized nonregenerated cellulose
ORC	Oxidized regenerated cellulose
PAI-1	Plasminogen activator inhibitor type 1
PAI-2	Plasminogen activator inhibitor-2
PE	Pulmonary embolism
PF4	Platelet factor 4
PFA-100	Platelet function analyzer-100
PGH_2	Prostaglandin H2
PGI_2	Prostacyclin, prostaglandin I2
pH	Potential of hydrogen
P-PRF	Pure platelet rich fibrin

PRF	Platelet-rich fibrin
PRP	Platelet-rich plasma
PT	Prothrombin time
rVIIa	Recombinant activated factor VIIa
SLE	Systemic Lupus Erythematosus
TA	Tranexamic acid
TAFI	Thrombin activatable fibrinolysis inhibitor
TF	Tissue factor
TFPI	Tissue factor pathway inhibitor
TGF_{β}	Transforming growth factor beta
tPA	Tissue plasminogen activator
TRALI	Transfusion-related acute lung injury
TT	Thrombin time
TTP	Thrombotic thrombocytopenic purpura
TXA_2	Thromboxane A2
UFH	Unfractionated heparin
UFH	Unfractioned heparin
uPA	Urokinase
VEGF	Vascular endothelial growth factor
VKAs	Vitamin K antagonists
VWD	von Willebrand disease
VWF	von Willebrand factor
WFH	World Federation of Hemophilia
WHO	World Health Organization

Part I

Introduction

Dental Management of Patients with Bleeding Disorders: General Considerations

1

Branislav V. Bajkin and Alison Dougall

Box 1.1 General Considerations Regarding Dental Treatment of Patients with Bleeding Disorders

1. *Proper diagnosis of bleeding tendency*
   - Medical history
   - Intraoral and extraoral examination
   - Laboratory testing
   - Consultation with patient's physician
2. *High importance of prevention of oral diseases*
3. *Prevention of postoperative complications*
   - Careful treatment planning
   - Inpatient/outpatient treatment depends on the risk of the procedure
   - Avoiding accidental injuries
   - LA considerations (safer techniques, use of LA with vasoconstrictor, slow application of LA)
   - Minimally traumatic surgical technique (avoid flap surgery, limit the number of teeth to be removed, consider sectioning of multi-rooted teeth)
   - Removal of all granulation tissues
   - Use of local hemostatic agents and measures to control oral bleeding

(continued)

B. V. Bajkin (✉)
University of Novi Sad, Faculty of Medicine, Dentistry Clinic of Vojvodina, Novi Sad, Serbia
e-mail: branislav.bajkin@mf.uns.ac.rs

A. Dougall
School of Dental Science, Trinity College Dublin, Dublin Dental University Hospital, Dublin, Ireland

B. V. Bajkin (ed.), *Bleeding Disorders and Dentistry*,
https://doi.org/10.1007/978-3-032-26713-9_1

Box 1.1 (continued)

- Provide a patient with postoperative instructions (avoid aspirin and other NSAIDs, soft and cold diet, phone number in case of an emergency) and regular follow-up

LA local anesthesia, *NSAIDs* nonsteroidal anti-inflammatory drugs

Box 1.2 Causes of Bleeding Following Dental Procedures

1. *Local causes of bleeding* (soft tissue trauma, sharp bone prominences, alveolar ridge fracture, foreign bodies, remaining granulation tissue, blood vessel injury)
2. *Bleeding disorders*
    - Vascular bleeding disorders
    - Disorders of platelet count and function
    - Coagulation disorders
    - Bleeding disorders in liver disease
    - Bleeding disorders in malignant diseases
3. *Use of antithrombotic agents*
    - Vitamin K antagonists
    - Direct oral anticoagulants
    - Antiplatelet agents
    - Heparin
4. *Incompliance with postoperative instructions* (mouth rinse, interference with the wound)

Oral diseases, such as caries and periodontal diseases (gingivitis and periodontitis), are among the most prevalent diseases in the population despite being highly preventable. The prevention of these diseases is of great importance in general population, but, considering possible complications, it is particularly important in patients with bleeding disorders.

Preventive measures should be taken at an early age and should include early preventive dental visits, motivation and training on proper oral hygiene, and pit and fissure sealing. Prevention of oral diseases and plaque control through regular checkups and dental hygiene should be performed during the whole life by using the proper toothbrushing technique with appropriate toothbrushes and fluoride toothpastes, antibacterial mouthwash solutions, dental floss, interdental brushes, and water jet devices. Regular dental checkups and periodic removal of soft and hard deposits from the teeth are of utmost importance. Removing deposits from the teeth not only prevents the onset of caries lesions and gum diseases but also reduces gingival inflammation, thus preventing gingival bleeding. The results of some studies indicate a higher incidence of caries and periodontal diseases in patients with bleeding disorders, which is mainly related to the fear of bleeding during toothbrushing or dental anxiety in these patients [1].

Dental management of patients with bleeding disorders primarily involves the prevention of oral and dental diseases and prevention of postoperative bleeding in cases when an operative dental procedure is needed. Any invasive dental procedure requires thorough planning and consultation with the patient's physician. The treatment should be scheduled in the morning and at the beginning of the workweek, so there would be enough time for patient's postoperative monitoring. The risk of postoperative bleeding mainly depends on the extent of a surgical procedure and the severity of a bleeding disorder. Depending on the risk of bleeding, the dental surgery can be done as an inpatient, a day case care, or outpatient procedure.

Prevention of postoperative bleeding begins with taking a patient's medical history which may reveal the following [2]:

1. Prolonged and extensive bleeding after previous tooth extractions, surgery, or traumas
2. Spontaneous bleeding (epistaxis, skin bruises, meno- and metrorrhagia in females)
3. The need for blood transfusion and the circumstances that led to it
4. Taking blood thinners (anticoagulant or antiplatelet therapy)
5. Liver diseases (jaundice, hepatitis, hepatocellular tumor)
6. Malignant diseases and blood diseases
7. Family history related to hereditary coagulopathies

Intraoral inspection may reveal the presence of gingival or oral mucosal bleeding in the form of petechia, ecchymosis, and hematoma (Fig. 1.1a, b). Similar bleeding manifestations can be observed on the skin (Figs. 1.1c and 1.2).

Laboratory testing is mandatory for the proper diagnosis of any bleeding disorder. Standard laboratory tests for assessing hemostatic function are bleeding time (BT), prothrombin time (PT), activated partial thromboplastin time (aPTT), platelet count, and fibrinogen (see Chap. 3). If necessary, some additional laboratory tests may be taken, such as determination of concentration of factor VIII (FVIII), factor IX (FIX), or von Willebrand factor (VWF), in case of hemophilia A, hemophilia B, or von Willebrand disease (VWD).

During the dental treatment, any accidental injury should be prevented. Accidental injury can happen during many dental procedures such as intraoral radiography, use of suction devices, removal of cotton rolls, removal of impressions, etc. Restorative dental procedures and root canal treatment are not considered as high-risk bleeding procedures. Matrix bands and wooden wedges should be placed carefully in order to avoid soft tissue trauma. Caution is necessary in cases of subgingival caries removal or subgingival scaling in persons with a severe bleeding disorder such as hemophilia. Prosthodontic and orthodontic treatments are considered safe as all measures are taken to prevent soft tissue injury.

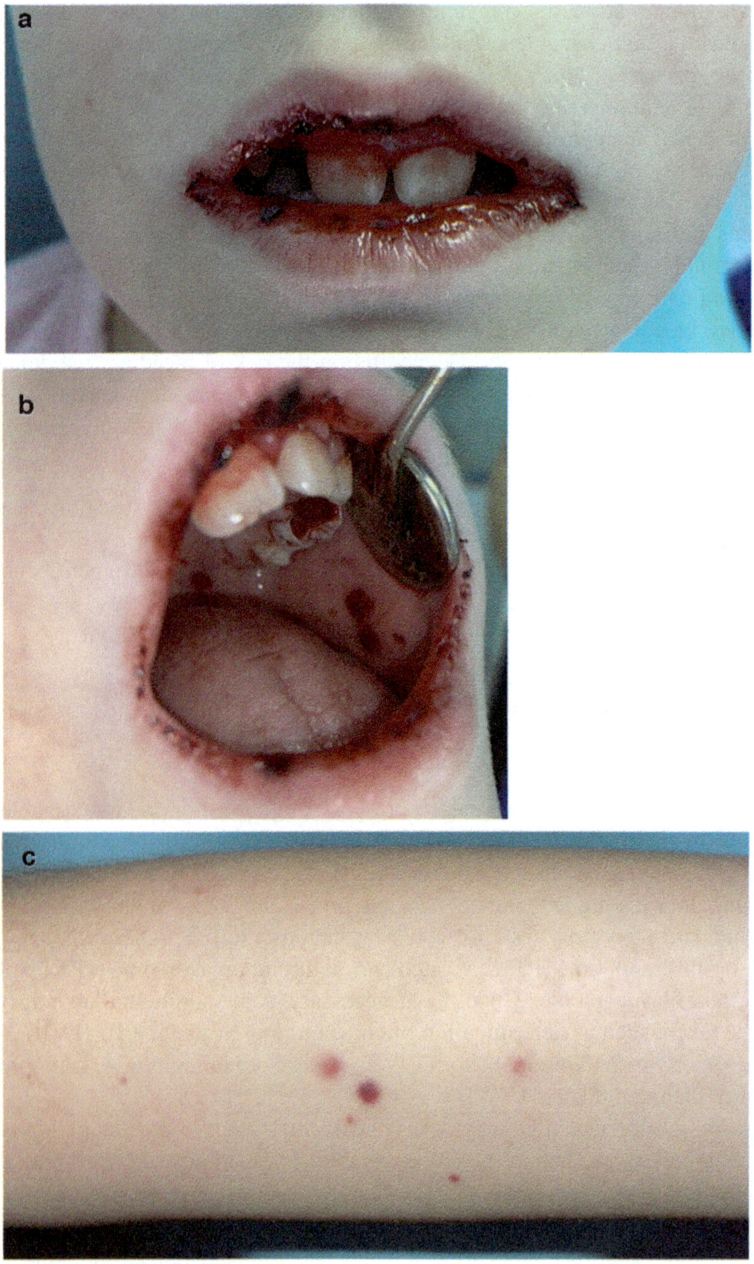

Fig. 1.1 (**a**, **b**) Intraoral findings in a child with thrombocytopenia (**c**) Skin lesions in a child with thrombocytopenia shown in Fig. 1.1a, b

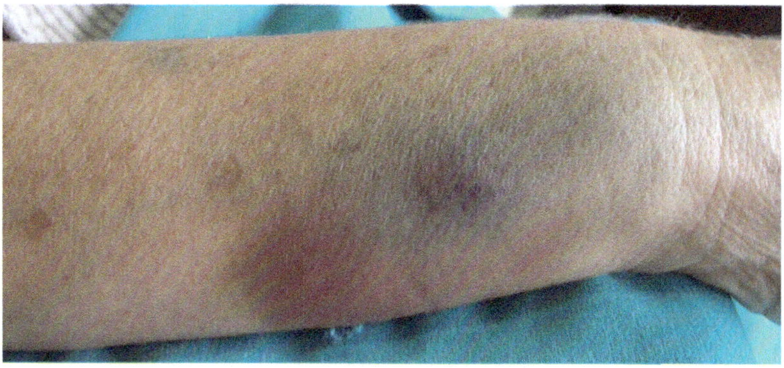

Fig. 1.2 Subcutaneous hematoma as a consequence of vitamin K antagonist therapy overdose

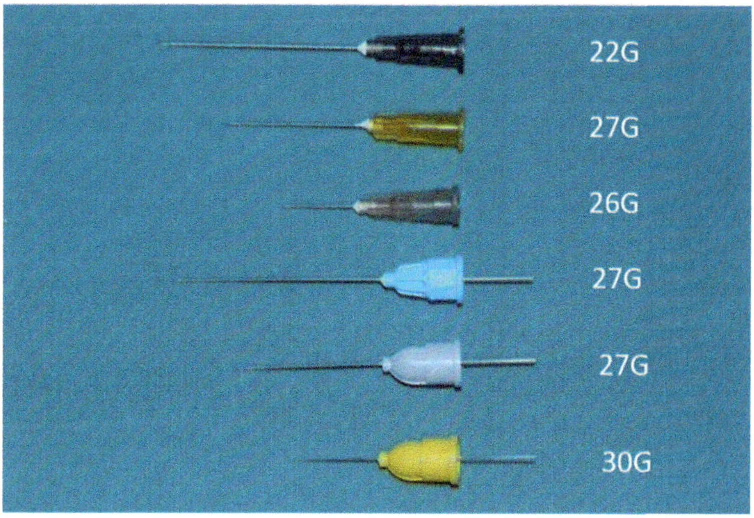

Fig. 1.3 Different needle gauges used for the administration of local anesthesia in dentistry

Minimally invasive dental techniques should be used. Preference should be given to safer local anesthesia techniques. Local infiltration and intraligamentary anesthesia are less likely to provoke bleeding complications compared to block anesthetic techniques. The use of cartridge syringes and needles with smaller diameter is recommended (Fig. 1.3). Multiple infiltrations of local anesthetics should be avoided as known of causing greater trauma of soft tissue (Figs. 1.4 and 1.5). Due to possible airway obstruction, in patients with severe bleeding disorders, such as those with hemophilia and VWD type 3, inferior alveolar nerve block (IANB) and sublingual infiltration are not recommended without factor replacement therapy. The use of local anesthetics with adrenaline reduces the risk of intraoperative bleeding. Aspiration and slow application of an anesthetic are mandatory to minimize soft tissue trauma. After IANB, the patients should be advised to be careful not to cause

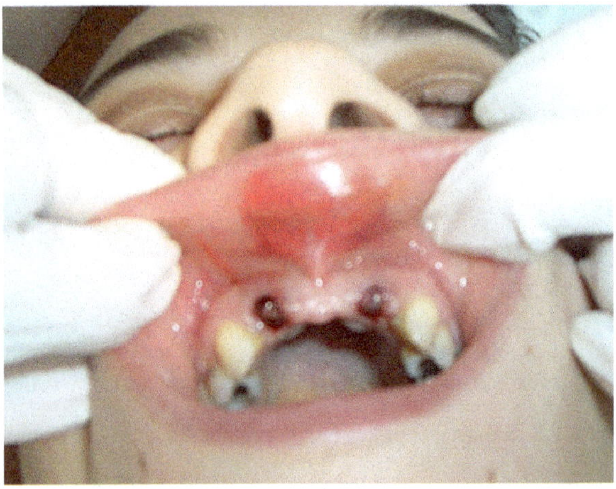

Fig. 1.4 Postanesthetic hematoma of the upper lip in a patient with idiopathic thrombocytopenic purpura (platelet count $<30 \times 10^9$/L)

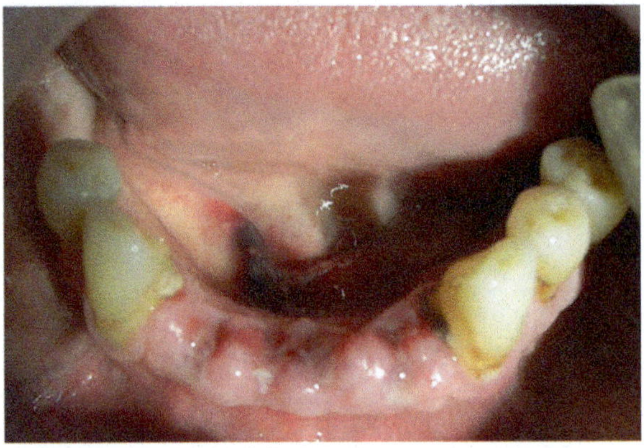

Fig. 1.5 Postanesthetic hematoma of the floor of the mouth following multiple local anesthetic infiltrations into the lingual sulcus in a patient on vitamin K antagonist therapy

self-injury by biting their lip or tongue due to temporary loss of sensation in these areas. The use of computer-controlled systems for applying local anesthetics may have advantages in patients with bleeding disorders.

Oral surgery should be performed with minimal trauma. Dentoalveolar procedures, such as tooth extraction, dental implant placement, and periodontal surgical procedures, are of special interest. It is estimated that the risk of bleeding during implant placement is similar to that during single tooth extraction. When extracting multirooted teeth, root separation should be considered. Releasing incisions and wide flaps should be avoided. If a bone removal is necessary, it should be done to the minimal extent and only as much as required. Granulation tissue should be carefully and completely removed from the extraction socket as it can be the cause of postoperative bleeding. Primary closure of the extraction wound can help in stabilization and protection of the blood clot and should always be done when the procedure does not require additional soft tissue manipulation. Bleeding after periodontal surgery can be difficult to treat because of a large bleeding surface area and a very limited possibility for applying local hemostatic agents.

The choice of local hemostatic agent depends on many factors including the type of dental or oral surgical procedure (tooth extraction or some other dentoalveolar or periodontal surgical procedure), previous experience of a dentist/surgeon, and costs and availability of these agents on the market (see Chap. 27). Along with the use of local hemostatic agents and wound suturing, gauze compression of the wound immediately after the procedure is highly important for achieving local hemostasis and initial stabilization of the blood clot.

Thorough postoperative instructions given to patients as well as good compliance with given recommendations are of great importance for the postoperative bleeding prevention. Patients should be advised to be on a soft and cold diet, not to spit, suck, and rinse their mouth, to avoid smoking and to gently brush their teeth for the first few days. Paracetamol or selective cyclooxygenase 2 inhibitors (COX-2 inhibitors) are considered the analgesics of choice in patients with bleeding disorders. Acetylsalicylic acid and other nonsteroidal anti-inflammatory drugs (NSAIDs) should be avoided due to antiplatelet effect and aggressive action on gastric mucosa. Patients should be provided with clear instructions what to do in case of postoperative bleeding and who to contact if the bleeding does not cease.

It is estimated that bleeding occurs in 0.2–3.3% of cases after oral surgical procedures in patients who do not have a bleeding disorder, while in those with bleeding disorders, it occurs in 8.6–32.1% of cases [3, 4]. Postoperative bleeding can be caused by local factors or systemic conditions such as bleeding disorder or a drug that affects coagulation or platelet function. The most common local causes of bleeding after tooth extraction are excessive operative trauma, particularly to oral soft tissues, irritation of the soft tissue by residual sharp bone edges, inflammation at the extraction site, fracture of the alveolar ridge or maxillary tuberosity (Fig. 1.6a, b), foreign body, granulation tissue left in the extraction wound, and injury of a major blood vessel in the oral cavity (Fig. 1.7). Removal of a benign lesion of vascular origin (Fig. 1.8a, b) or dental procedure in the region of arteriovenous malformation (Fig. 1.9a, b) requires extreme caution. Bleeding is often caused by poor compliance with the postoperative instructions, such as mouth rinsing or any additional trauma or interference with the wound throughout the process of healing. Increased salivary fibrinolytic activity caused by local inflammation should not be forgotten as a potential cause of bleeding.

It is a wrong presumption that postoperative bleeding in patients with a bleeding disorder is necessarily caused by the disorder itself. Local causes of bleeding should be eliminated first. Dental examination and the use of local hemostatic agents are necessary prior to systemic measures for bleeding control in these patients.

Bleeding after oral surgical procedures can be normal or excessive, ranging from mild and moderate to severe, posing a threat to the patient's life. Mild bleeding can be easily controlled by local compression. Moderate bleeding requires wound revision and application of additional hemostatic agents and measures. Severe bleeding may require hospitalization, use of systemic measures, and blood transfusion [5]. Bleeding on the floor of the mouth is considered to be particularly serious because of potential airway obstruction.

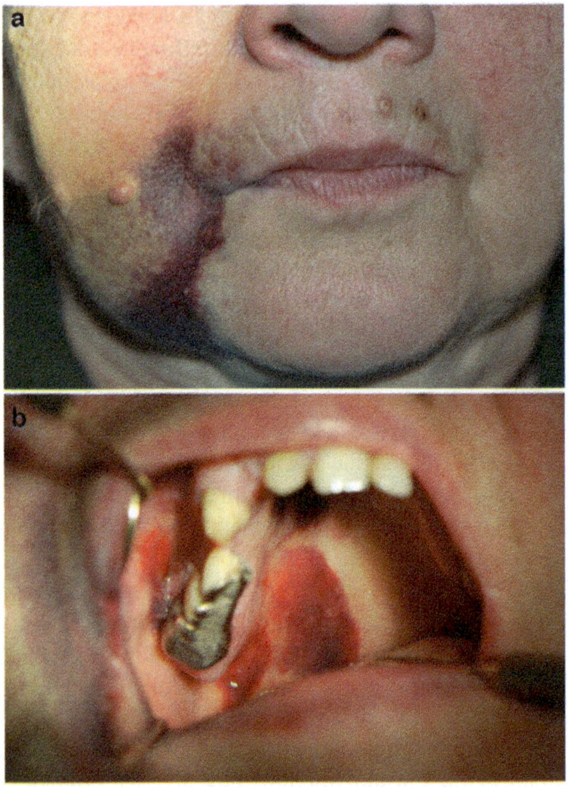

Fig. 1.6 (**a**) Facial hematoma resulting from maxillary tuberosity fracture (**b**) Intraoral hematoma secondary to fracture of the maxillary tuberosity in the patient shown in Fig. 1.6a

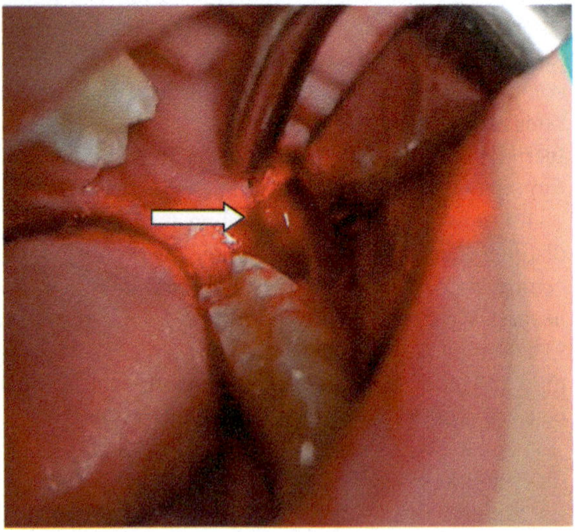

Fig. 1.7 Hemorrhage due to injury of the retromolar artery during surgical extraction of the mandibular third molar

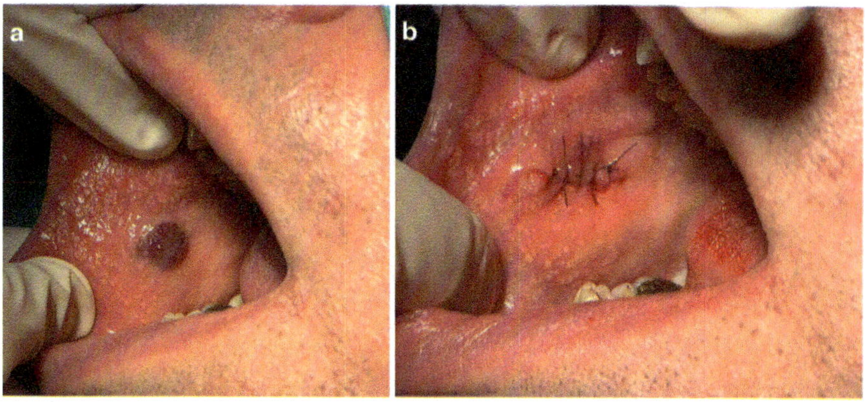

Fig. 1.8 (**a**) Hemangioma of the buccal mucosa (**b**) Postoperative wound following removal of the hemangioma

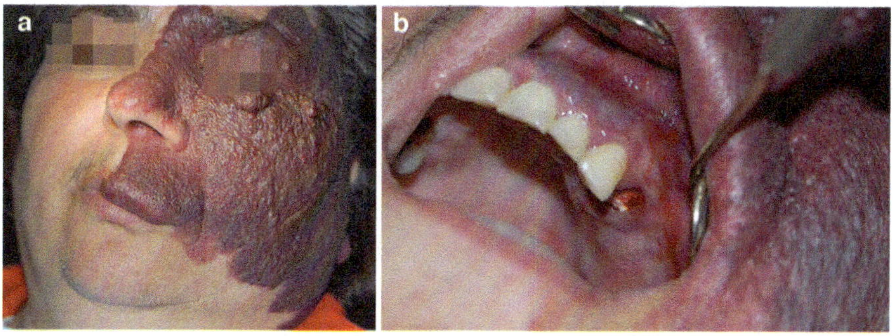

Fig. 1.9 (**a**) Facial vascular malformation (**b**) Tooth extraction in the region of an vascular malformation with application of a collagen-based local hemostatic agent into the extraction socket

References

1. Gupta A, Epstein JB, Cabay RJ. Bleeding disorders of importance in dental care and related patient management. J Can Dent Assoc. 2007;73:77–83.
2. Hupp JR, Yeung A. Preoperative health status evaluation. In: Hupp JR, Ellis III E, Tucker MR, editors. Contemporary oral and maxillofacial surgery. 7th ed. Elsevier; 2019. p. 2–19.
3. Reich W, Kriwalsky MS, Wolf HH, Schubert J. Bleeding complications after oral surgery in outpatients with compromised haemostasis: incidence and management. Oral Maxillofac Surg. 2009;13:73–7.
4. De Padua V, Romeo U, Santoro C, Bosco R, Baldacci E, Ferretti A, Malaspina F, Mazzucconi MG, Gaglioti D. Dental invasive procedures in von Willebrand disease outpatients treated with high purity FVIII/VWF complex concentrate (Fanhdi®): experience of a single center. Heliyon. 2020;6(2):e03426.
5. Lockhart PB, Gibson J, Pond SH, Leitch J. Dental management considerations for the patient with an acquired coagulopathy. Part 1: Coagulopathies from systemic disease. Br Dent J. 2003;195(8):439–45.

Part II

Normal Hemostasis and Coagulation

Fundamentals of Normal Hemostasis

2

Branislav V. Bajkin and Ivana Urosevic

Hemostasis is a term that relates to all physiological processes that maintain blood in a liquid state and allow blood flow within blood vessels. It also relates to all the mechanisms that prevent blood outflow in normal conditions or leads to cessation of bleeding in case of a vessel damage. It is a complex defense mechanism that protects the integrity of blood vessels. Normal hemostasis is based on the interaction of blood vessels, platelets, coagulation factors, and the fibrinolytic system.

In the physiological conditions and when there is no damage of the blood vessel wall, these components are in a mutually neutral state and allow normal blood flow through the vessels, thus preventing the formation of thrombus. There is a balance between procoagulant factors on one side and natural coagulation inhibitors and fibrinolytic system on the other. When an injury occurs, the endothelium and subendothelium of the injured blood vessel initiate a complex process that leads to cessation of bleeding at the site of injury, while the existing balance in the rest of the body is maintained. The coagulation process stops at a certain point, so that there is no obstruction in blood flow at the site of injury.

Normal hemostasis represents a balance between prothrombotic and anticoagulant processes. There are five components of hemostasis:

- Vascular
- Platelets
- Coagulation factors
- Coagulation inhibitors (natural inhibitors)
- Fibrinolysis or clot dissolution

B. V. Bajkin (✉)
University of Novi Sad, Faculty of Medicine, Dentistry Clinic of Vojvodina, Novi Sad, Serbia
e-mail: branislav.bajkin@mf.uns.ac.rs

I. Urosevic
University of Novi Sad, Faculty of Medicine, University Clinical Center of Vojvodina, Clinic of Hematology, Novi Sad, Serbia

B. V. Bajkin (ed.), *Bleeding Disorders and Dentistry*,
https://doi.org/10.1007/978-3-032-26713-9_2

Considering the importance of each of these components, their role will be discussed separately in the following section of this chapter.

2.1 Blood Vessels

Hemostasis is a dynamic process that initially involves blood vessel wall and platelets. After injury of a blood vessel, vasoconstriction that occurs induces the reduced blood flow through the injured vessel and decreased blood outflow. Slower blood flow initiates adhesion and activation of platelets, which further triggers the coagulation cascade. Vasoconstriction is primarily a result of myogenic spasm [1]. Vasoconstriction of arteries and arterioles is under neural control, while the constriction of smaller blood vessels, such as capillaries, is mediated by humoral and local factors. Vasoconstriction is enhanced by mediators that interact with smooth muscles in the vessel wall. These mediators are released from platelets and endothelial cells. The most important are thromboxane A2 (TXA_2), endothelin, prostaglandin H2 (PGH_2), adenosine-diphosphate (ADP), and serotonin (5-HT) [2, 3]. The initial vasoconstriction is followed by vasodilation, which usually does not pose a risk in terms of rebleeding, except in patients with hemorrhagic diathesis.

Endothelial cells line the blood vessels. They come into contact with the blood and function as a barrier between the blood and subendothelial tissue. The physiological roles of the endothelium are extensive. It controls vascular permeability, the movement of nutrients and biologically active molecules, and the interaction of blood cells with the vessel wall. It also participates in angiogenesis and the inflammatory response [4]. Additionally, the endothelium plays a crucial role in preventing thrombus formation. Along with collagen, elastin, and fibronectin—components found in the subendothelium—the endothelium maintains the integrity of the blood vessel wall.

The intact endothelial smooth surface has antithrombogenic properties, supported by its secretory function and by binding of antithrombin (AT), a natural anticoagulant on the surface of the endothelium. AT is synthesized in the liver and circulates in the plasma. It inactivates thrombin and activates coagulation factors (FIXa, FXa, FXIa, and FXIIa). The endothelial cells express thrombomodulin, another anticoagulant protein that binds thrombin. Tissue plasminogen activator (tPA), prostaglandin I2 (prostacyclin, PGI_2), and nitric oxide (NO) are synthesized in endothelium. tPa converts circulating plasminogen into plasmin, which has a fibrinolytic action, while prostacyclin and NO are vasodilators and inhibitors of platelet aggregation [2, 3, 5, 6].

In contrast to the antithrombogenic properties of the intact endothelial surface, endothelial damage changes the surface to prothrombogenic and leads to the activation of complex mechanisms that initiate bleeding cessation by platelet adhesion and activation, coagulation, and inhibition of fibrinolysis. Endothelium has an active role in hemostasis. Von Willebrand factor (VWF) is synthesized in endothelial cells. VWF affects platelet adhesion at the site of injury by binding to collagen and receptors on the platelet membrane (Fig. 2.1). A strong stimulus for initiation of bleeding cessation is the contact of blood and exposed subendothelium. Collagen, tissue factor (TF), and VWF have a significant role in this process [2, 6]. Platelet adhesion and aggregation are initiated by the interaction of platelet membrane receptors,

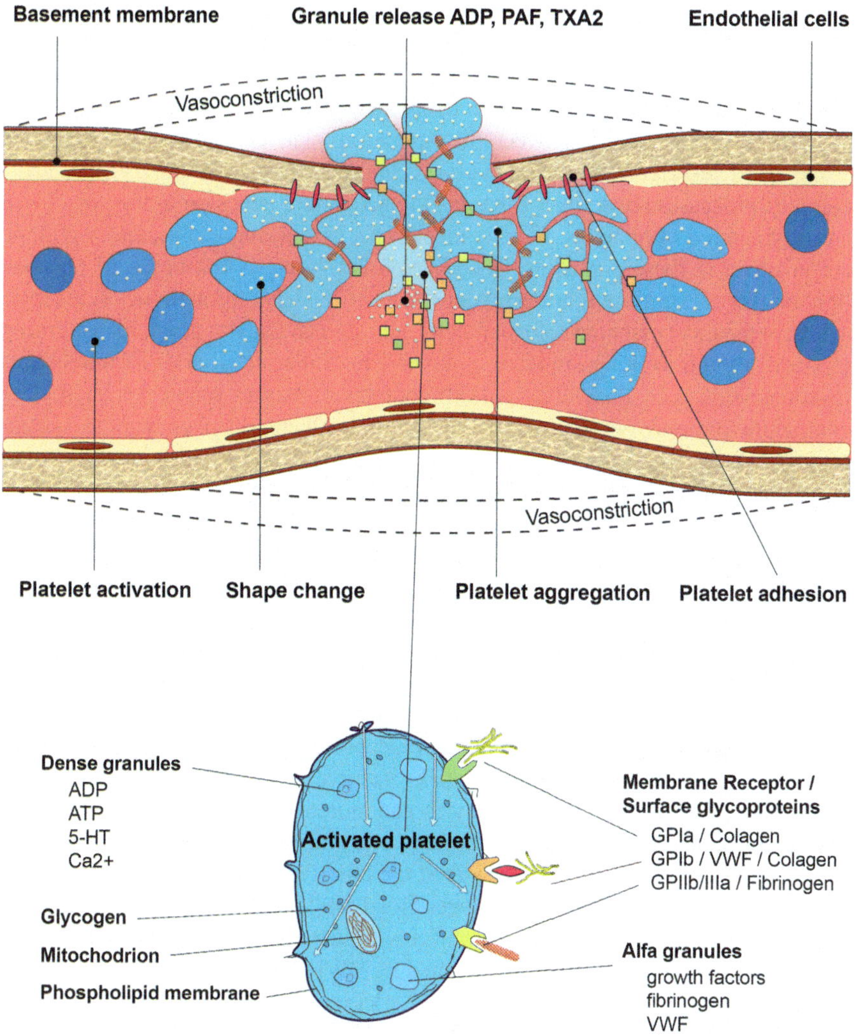

Fig. 2.1 (**a**) Platelet adhesion, activation, and aggregation. (**b**) Activated platelet

VWF, and exposed collagen at the site of injury. Platelet activation is also influenced by reduced blood flow due to vasoconstriction but also by the inflammatory processes in the endothelium [4].

2.2 Platelets

Platelets are small (2–3 μm), anucleate, disc-shaped cells. They are formed in the bone marrow from megakaryocytes. A normal platelet count in blood is 150–450 × 10^9/L. The main regulator of platelet production is thrombopoietin, a hormone produced by the liver and kidneys. Thrombopoietin binds to receptors on megakaryocytes, stimulating platelet production. Two-thirds of the total number of platelets are in circulation, while the rest is stored in the spleen. The average lifespan of platelets is 7–10 days. Platelets are removed from circulation in the spleen and liver mainly through the tissue macrophage system [1, 2, 4, 6].

There is no interaction between the circulating platelets and intact endothelium of the blood vessels. When a blood vessel is injured, subendothelium is exposed and complex processes are activated that lead to activation, adhesion to the vessel wall, and aggregation of platelets. Platelet membrane, cytoplasm, and secretory granules are involved in these processes. The platelet membrane is composed of phospholipid bilayer and transmembrane glycoproteins (GP). Glycoproteins act as receptors and have the most essential role in platelet adhesion and aggregation. Platelet receptors activate intracellular signaling pathways by initiating a series of intracellular reactions (Fig. 2.1). Platelet cytoplasm contains numerous molecules such as (1) contractile proteins actin, myosin, and thrombosthenin; (2) enzymatic systems capable of synthesizing adenosine-diphosphate (ADP), adenosine triphosphate (ATP), and prostaglandins; (3) fibrin-stabilizing factor; and (4) growth factors [1].

Platelet hemostatic function involves activation, adhesion, and aggregation. The initial steps of platelet activation and adhesion occur after a blood vessel injury, as VWF binds to the receptor complex GPIb-IX-V (GPIb), and when subendothelial collagen directly contacts receptors on the platelet membrane. The complex process of platelet activation and aggregation is facilitated by VWF, thrombin, TXA2, 5-HT, epinephrine, and ADP [2, 5, 7, 8].

Upon blood vessel injury, platelets adhere to the injury site through a process involving exposed collagen, glycoprotein receptors on the platelet membrane, and VWF. VWF is a glycoprotein that remains inactive in circulation. It is synthesized in endothelial cells and megakaryocytes and stored in α-granules. VWF binds to both collagen and the GpIb receptor, acting as a link between exposed collagen and platelets. This reaction can be considered the initial event in platelet adhesion. The adhesion process is facilitated by slower blood flow and the movement of platelets themselves, which promotes easier contact with subendothelial tissue. In addition to the collagen and platelet binding mediated by VWF, collagen also binds directly to platelets via integrin α2β1 (GpIa/IIa) and GpVI receptors [2, 5, 6, 8]. Adhesion and subsequent aggregation are further influenced by other mediators present in the subendothelium and platelet granules, such as fibronectin, laminin, thrombospondin, and vitronectin.

Platelets have two forms of secretory granules that release their contents upon the platelet activation (Fig. 2.1b). Molecules stored in α-granules have a role in hemostasis, immune and inflammatory response, and wound healing. These granules contain platelet factor 4 (PF4), α-thromboglobulin, VWF, coagulation factors (FI, FV, FXI, and FXIII), protein S, plasminogen activator inhibitor (PAI-1), growth factors, thrombospondin, fibronectin, and others. 5-HT, ADP, ATP, and calcium are stored in dense granules [2]. The released granule content further accelerates platelet adhesion aggregation and mutual interaction of platelets. Activated platelets via the cyclooxygenase 1 (COX-1) pathway synthesize TXA_2 (Fig. 2.2), which promotes vasoconstriction and accelerates platelet adhesion and aggregation [5, 8].

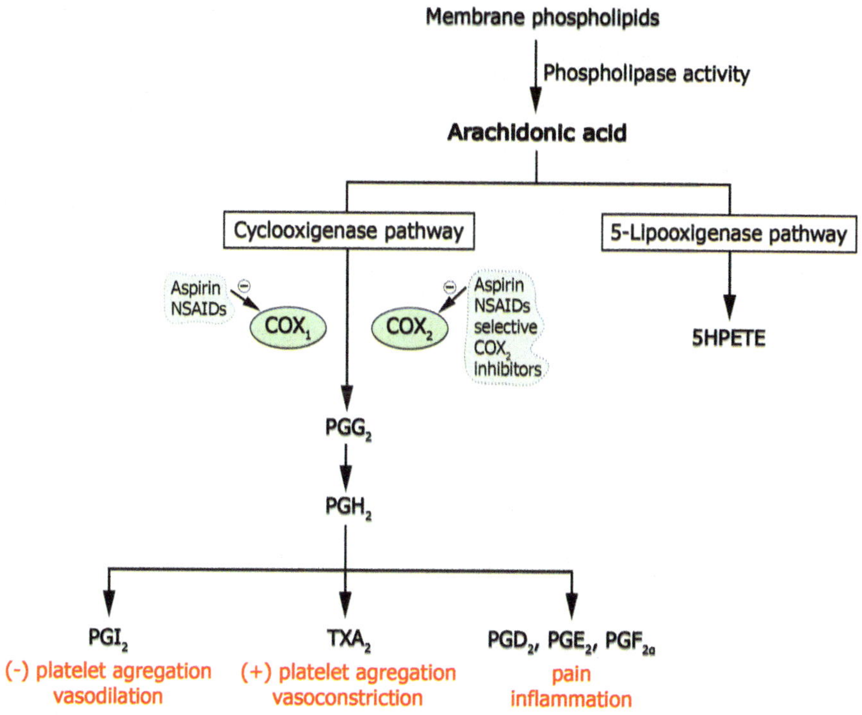

Fig. 2.2 Arachidonic acid pathway
COX2, cyclooxigenase-2 pathway; COX1, cyclooxigenase-1 pathway; NSAIDs, nonsteroidal anti-inflammatory drugs; PGG_2, prostaglandin G2; PGH_2, prostaglandin H2; PGI_2, prostaglandin I2; TXA_2, thromboxane A2; PGD_2, prostaglandin D2; PGE_2, prostaglandin E2; $PGF_{2\alpha}$, prostaglandin F2α; 5HPETE, 5-hydroperoxyicosatetraenoic acid

Adhesion is accompanied by a change in platelet shape under the influence of contractile proteins and the initiation of procoagulant mechanisms that further lead to platelet activation. Platelet adhesion initiates intracellular signaling pathways that activate the GpIIb/IIIa receptor (integrin αIIbβ3). GpIIb/IIIa is the most common GP receptor on the platelet surface and remains inactive under normal physiological conditions.

Aggregation or the sticking of platelets to each other is caused by the binding of activated GpIIb/IIIa receptors on the membranes of neighboring platelets with the involvement of fibrinogen. Fibrinogen, converted into fibrin, stabilizes the platelet plug. The binding of VWF to the GpIIb/IIIa receptor also promotes platelet aggregation [2, 7, 8]. By adhesion and aggregation, platelet mass is increased at the site of injury, forming a basis for initiating the coagulation process.

Platelet plug formation is also called primary hemostasis, while secondary hemostasis refers to the coagulation phase and the formation of a fibrin clot. The blood vessel wall and platelets participate in primary hemostasis. Platelets, along with coagulation factors, are involved in secondary hemostasis. The activated platelet surface leads to the activation of coagulation factors, while TF, also known as thromboplastin, initiates the external coagulation pathway.

Besides their crucial role in forming blood clots after blood vessel injury, platelets also play a key role in pathological processes that lead to thrombus formation in arterial and venous vessels, which underpin many cardiovascular diseases and are among the most common causes of death. The most common signs of arterial thrombosis are myocardial infarction and ischemic cerebrovascular attack, while symptoms of venous thrombosis include deep vein thrombosis and pulmonary embolism. Although arterial and venous thrombosis differ in their biological mechanisms, they share similar risk factors [9]. Arterial thrombi mainly form through platelet interactions with one another and with the damaged endothelium of blood vessels. The rupture of an atherosclerotic plaque followed by platelet adhesion and aggregation is the primary cause of arterial thrombosis. Virchow's triad describes risk factors for venous thrombosis, but today more emphasis is placed on hypercoagulability and venous stasis compared to endothelial injury [10].

2.3 Overview of the Coagulation System

Coagulation is a complex process that involves the activation and interaction of numerous coagulation factors resulting in the formation of a fibrin clot. Coagulation has traditionally been described as a cascade model, or a series of reactions that follow one after the other in the intrinsic, extrinsic, and common coagulation pathways, resulting in the formation of a fibrin clot. The cell-based model of coagulation is currently accepted as the model that better describes coagulation process in vivo. This model also provides more precise explanation of cellular and enzymatic hemostatic reactions as well as hemostatic disorders.

In this chapter, both models of coagulation, cascade, and cell base have been presented along with the overview of coagulation factors and natural anticoagulants.

2.3.1 Coagulation Factors

There are 12 coagulation factors that are designated by Roman numerals according to the generally accepted recommendations of the International Committee for the Standardization of the Nomenclature of Blood Clotting Factors from 1954 to 1958. The letter "F" in front and the small letter "a" after the Roman numeral specify factor and activated factor, respectively [1, 11]. Coagulation factors circulate in the plasma in an inactive form. Most of them are proenzymes, which are activated by proteolysis from their zymogens in coagulation cascade reaction. The presence of cofactors is necessary for the activation of some of those proenzymes (Table 2.1).

Fibrinogen (FI) is a protein that is primarily synthesized in hepatocytes and circulates in the plasma. The final phase of coagulation is the conversion of fibrinogen into fibrin (FIa) mediated by the thrombin. The polymerized fibrin, together with

Table 2.1 Coagulation factors

Factor	Synonym(s)	Site of synthesis	Main function	Coagulation pathway
FI	Fibrinogen	Liver	Forming fibrin clot	Common
FII	Prothrombin	Liver; vitamin K-dependent factor	Fibrinogen transformation into fibrin	Common
FIII	Tissue factor; thromboplastin	Subendothelium; perivascular tissues	Coagulation initiation; FVII activation	Extrinsic
FIV	Calcium	Stored in bones; food intake	Cofactor for FII, FIX, FX, FXI	Intrinsic and extrinsic
FV	Proaccelerin; labile factor	Liver; megakaryocytes	Cofactor for FII	Common
FVII	Prothrombin conversion accelerator; proconvertin; stable factor	Liver; vitamin K-dependent factor	Initiation of extrinsic pathway with FIII; FX activation	Extrinsic
FVIII	Antihemophilic factor A; antihemophilic factor; antihemophilic globulin	Liver	Cofactor for FIX	Intrinsic
FIX	Antihemophilic factor B; plasma thromboplastin component; Christmas factor	Liver; vitamin K-dependent factor	FX activation	Intrinsic
F X	Stuart-Prower factor; Stuart factor	Liver; vitamin K-dependent factor	Prothrombin transformation into thrombin	Common
FXI	Plasma thromboplastin antecedent; antihemophilic factor C	Liver; megakaryocytes	FIX activation	Intrinsic
FXII	Hageman factor	Liver	FXI activation	Intrinsic
FXIII	Fibrin-stabilizing factor	Liver; megakaryocytes	Fibrin clot stabilization	Common
	Prekallikrein; Fletcher factor	Liver	Acceleration of FXI activation by FXII	Intrinsic
	High-molecular-weight kininogen; Fitzgerald factor	Liver	FXI activation by FXII	Intrinsic

platelets, forms a blood clot. In addition, fibrinogen is also involved in platelet aggregation by binding to the GPIIb/IIIa receptor on the platelet membrane.

Prothrombin (FII) is synthesized in the liver, and it is one of the four vitamin K-dependent coagulation factors (FII, FVII, FIX, and FX). The active form of this factor is thrombin which converts fibrinogen into fibrin. Thrombin also affects the activation of platelets and FV, FVIII, FIX, and FXIII.

Tissue factor (TF) is found in subendothelial cells. It is also known as coagulation factor III (FIII) or tissue thromboplastin. After blood vessel injury, TF initiates coagulation.

FIV and FV are cofactors. Serum ionized calcium (FIV) is essential to the coagulation process, participating in activation of many clotting factors (FII, FIX, FX,

FXI, and FXII) in all three coagulation pathways. FV (proaccelerin) is synthesized in the liver and, together with calcium, participates in the conversion of prothrombin (FII) into thrombin.

FVII is a vitamin K-dependent factor that is synthesized in the liver. After a blood vessel injury, together with TF (F III), it initiates the extrinsic coagulation pathway.

FVIII is also known as antihemophilic factor A. The lack of this factor is the cause of hemophilia A. FVIII is synthesized in the liver sinusoidal endothelial cells, and it circulates in the plasma being bound to VWF. As a cofactor, together with calcium, it activates FX.

FIX or Christmas factor is a vitamin K-dependent coagulation factor synthesized in the liver. The deficiency of this factor is the cause of hemophilia B. It participates in the intrinsic coagulation pathway.

FX, FXI, and FXII are synthesized in the liver. FX is a vitamin K-dependent factor that catalyzes the conversion of prothrombin (FII) to thrombin in the common coagulation pathway. FXI and FXII act in the intrinsic coagulation pathway.

FXIII is a fibrin-stabilizing factor. It is activated by thrombin. After the conversion of fibrinogen to fibrin, FXIII strengthens fibrin clot by cross-linking fibrin chains [1, 5, 11].

In addition to coagulation factors, other enzymes also play a significant role in the coagulation process. The most important ones are prekallikrein (*Fletcher* factor) and high-molecular-weight kininogen (HMWK). Prekallikrein is a precursor of kallikrein, an enzyme that cleaves HMWK, releasing the vasoactive peptide bradykinin. The kallikrein-kinin system has several important functions in the body such as contact activation of the intrinsic coagulation pathway, inflammation, blood pressure control, pain, and cell proliferation [1, 5, 11].

2.3.2 Cascade Model of Coagulation

The cascade (waterfall) model describes coagulation as it happens in vitro, in the laboratory. Coagulation cascade is the series of enzymatic reactions that result in activation of coagulation factors. Coagulation cascade is divided into extrinsic and intrinsic pathways. Both pathways converge to form the common pathway, which begins with the activation of FX (Fig. 2.3).

The extrinsic coagulation pathway is also known as TF pathway because it begins with the initiation of coagulation by TF. It requires external factor for the initiation. After a blood vessel injury, exposed TF binds and activates FVIIa, forming the complex TF-FVIIa. This complex activates FX into FXa. FXa in the presence of calcium ions and FVa forms the FXa-FVa prothrombinase complex (strongly stimulated by platelet phospholipids) and converts prothrombin to thrombin in the common coagulation pathway. The extrinsic coagulation pathway is faster compared to the intrinsic pathway. Once formed, thrombin further accelerates its own generation and the intrinsic coagulation pathway by activating FVIII and FV.

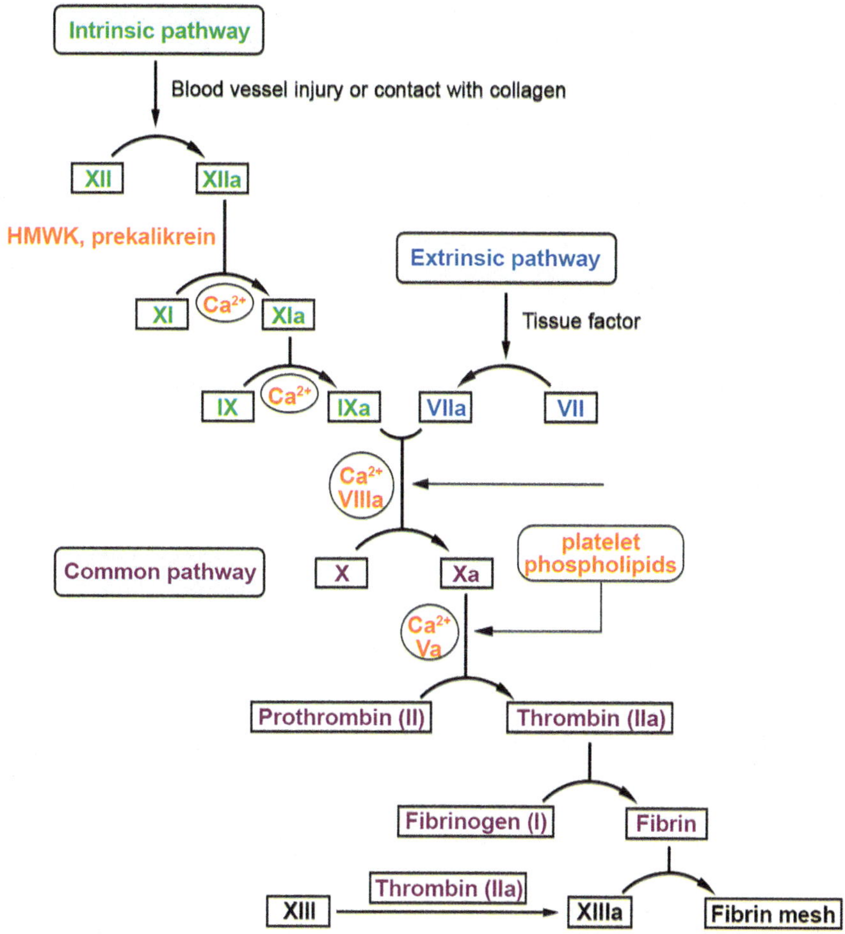

Fig. 2.3 Coagulation pathways

FVIII, FIX, FXI, and FXII participate in the intrinsic coagulation pathway, also known as the contact activation pathway. This pathway begins with the activation of factor FXII induced by contact with negatively charged surfaces. Exposed collagen from the injured blood vessel facilitates this activation. Activated platelets release platelet phospholipids (platelet factor 3) that activates intrinsic clotting factors. FXIIa further activates FXI in a reaction that involves HMWK and prekallikrein. FXIa activates FIX, which then in the presence of cofactor FVIII, calcium, and platelet phospholipid activates FX, leading to the formation of a prothrombin activator.

The common pathway begins with the formation of a prothrombin activator. Prothrombin activator is a complex of several activated coagulation factors. FXa, activated by the extrinsic or intrinsic pathway, in the presence of FVa, calcium ions, and platelet phospholipid converts prothrombin (FII) into thrombin. Thrombin cleaves fibrinogen (FI) into fibrin monomers. Fibrin monomers tend to spontaneously polymerize into fibrin fibers. Such polymers are weakly connected; thus, the initial fibrin clot is weak. FXIII activated by thrombin stabilizes fibrin fibers by creating covalent bonds and cross-linking them. This stabilizes fibrin clot. The blood clot subsequently retracts in a process initiated by platelets and extrudes most of the fluid, called serum [1, 5, 11].

2.3.3 Cellular Model of Hemostasis

Over time, it has become clear that the cascade model of coagulation does not fully and accurately describe what occurs during coagulation in vivo. Deficiencies in different coagulation factors do not produce the same clinical symptoms or bleeding tendencies. For example, the absence of FXII, prekallikrein, and HMWK does not relate to severe bleeding. Similarly, a deficiency in FXI is not always clinically evident as a severe bleeding disorder. In contrast, deficiency of FVIII or FIX is associated with severe bleeding tendencies. The lack of FVII is linked to severe clinical bleeding despite no abnormalities in the intrinsic pathway. It has also been observed that membrane phospholipids of certain cells—such as platelets, monocytes, and endothelial cells—play a significant role in coagulation. All of this has led to the development of a cell-based coagulation model. A brief overview of this model will be provided in the following text (Fig. 2.4).

According to current understandings, the extrinsic coagulation pathway is generally considered more dominant and initiates coagulation, while intrinsic pathway enhances the process. The extrinsic pathway is triggered by contact of perivascular tissue and circulating factors in plasma. TF exposed upon blood vessel injury rapidly binds FVII leading to its activation (FVIIa). The TF-FVIIa complex activates FX, directly but also indirectly through the activation of FIX. As a result of the interaction of FXa and cofactor FVa, a small amount of thrombin is produced at the TF-FVIIa complex. This phase of the cellular model of coagulation is called the initiation phase. The production of thrombin via the TF-FVIIa complex is a self-limiting reaction because it only takes place on the membranes of cells carrying TF. Further limitation is the rapid inactivation of FXa due to the action of antithrombin but also the action of the tissue factor pathway inhibitor (TFPI), a reversible inhibitor of the TF-FVIIa-FXa complex [1, 7, 11–13].

The created thrombin has multiple roles. It activates platelets, FV, FVIII, and FXI, which is called the amplification phase. Activation of FXI is not primarily triggered by the action of FXIIa, as presented in the cascade mechanism, but by the positive feedback reaction mediated by thrombin. For this reason, FXIa is more involved in amplification and propagation than in the initiation phase of coagulation [1, 7, 11–13]. The fact that the TF-FVIIa complex activates FIX has led to a different view of the coagulation process. It has been realized that there is a connection between the intrinsic and extrinsic coagulation pathways.

Considering that TFPI does not affect FIXa, this factor circulates in plasma and binds to the membrane of activated platelets. FVa, FVIIIa, FIXa, and FXIa also bind

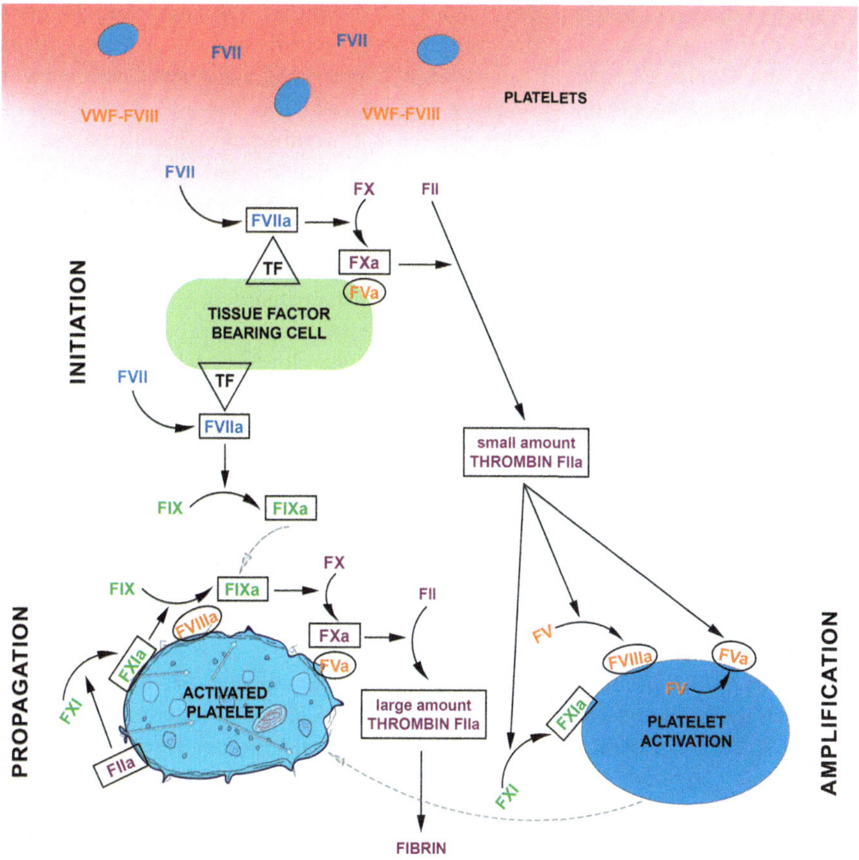

Fig. 2.4 Cell-based model of coagulation

to the membrane of activated platelets leading to the activation of FX and the production of a larger amount of thrombin on the surface of platelets. The generation of thrombin on the surface of platelets is called the propagation phase. Thrombin converts fibrinogen into fibrin and activates FXIII. The clot is then stabilized by covalent bonding of fibrin fibers under the influence of FXIIIa [1, 7, 8, 11–13].

It should be emphasized that the processes of initiation, amplification, and propagation are not separate; they occur concurrently and overlap with each other. The coagulation process ends with the formation of a blood clot containing platelets and fibrin.

2.3.4 Natural Anticoagulants

Under normal physiological conditions, there is a balance between procoagulant components (platelets, coagulation factors), anticoagulant components, and the fibrinolytic system. This balance maintains blood in a liquid state, allows blood flow within blood vessels, and prevents bleeding when a blood vessel is injured. If hemostasis becomes unbalanced, either bleeding or thrombosis may occur. Procoagulant components were described in the previous chapters, and this chapter will focus on anticoagulant components.

The smooth surface of the endothelium is antithrombogenic. Endothelial surface is covered by glycocalyx that prevents binding of platelets and coagulation factors. Endothelial cells also secrete PGI_2 and NO which are vasodilators and inhibitors of platelet aggregation [1]. The process of coagulation is self-limited due to quick binding of thrombin to fibrin fibers within the blood clot. In addition, natural anticoagulants play a significant role in maintaining the balance.

Natural anticoagulants are antithrombin, thrombomodulin, protein C and S, and TFPI. These substances inhibit the process of blood clot formation opposing either coagulation system or adhesion and aggregation of platelets (Fig. 2.5).

Antithrombin, also known as antithrombin III, is synthesized in the liver and endothelium. It is the main inhibitor of thrombin and FIXa, FXa, FXIa, and FXIIa. Heparin enhances antithrombin's activity by several hundred to several thousand times [1, 6].

Thrombomodulin is synthesized by endothelial cells. By binding thrombin to thrombomodulin, a complex is formed on the surface of the endothelium. This complex activates protein C. Bound thrombin is unable to activate platelets and convert fibrinogen into fibrin.

Protein C is a vitamin K-dependent natural anticoagulant. It is activated by thrombin-thrombomodulin complex on endothelial cells. It inactivates FVa and FVIIIa. Activated protein C also stimulates fibrinolysis. Protein S, whose synthesis also depends on vitamin K, is a nonenzymatic cofactor that enhances the effects of activated protein C.

TFPI is released from the endothelium. It neutralizes TF-FVIIa-FXa complex in extrinsic pathway of coagulation, as well as free FXa. The heparin-mediated release of TFPI may be of importance for anticoagulant effect of unfractionated and low molecular weight heparins [6, 7, 11].

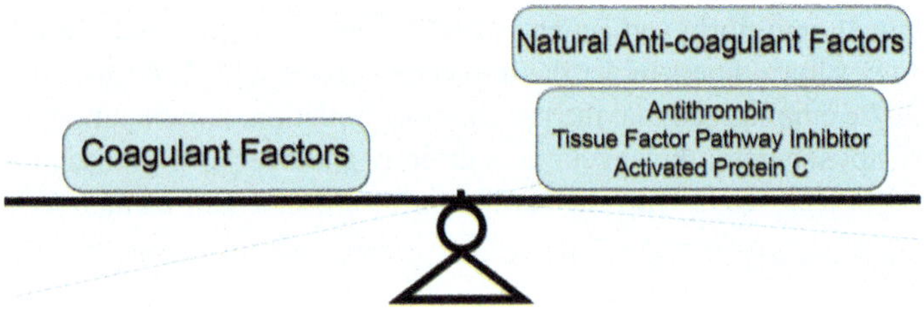

Fig. 2.5 Balance of normal coagulation

2.4 Fibrinolytic System

Upon a blood vessel injury, bleeding stops after formation of a blood clot. The fibrinolytic system is responsible for breaking down the blood clot to maintain the blood flow and allow wound healing. This is a physiological process, and it is along with coagulation a normal response to blood vessel damage. Fibrinolysis is the breakdown of fibrin under the action of plasmin. Plasmin originates from proenzyme plasminogen activated by plasminogen activators. Plasminogen is produced in the liver and released into circulation as an inactive plasmin precursor. During the process of blood clot formation, plasminogen is incorporated into the structure of coagulum by binding to fibrinogen and fibrin. tPa released from the endothelial cells also binds to fibrin and activates plasminogen incorporated in a blood clot, transforming it into active enzyme plasmin. Plasmin breaks down both fibrinogen and fibrin by cleaving them at multiple sites, and fibrin degradation products are released (Fig. 2.6). D-dimer is a fibrin degradation product and marker of fibrinolysis.

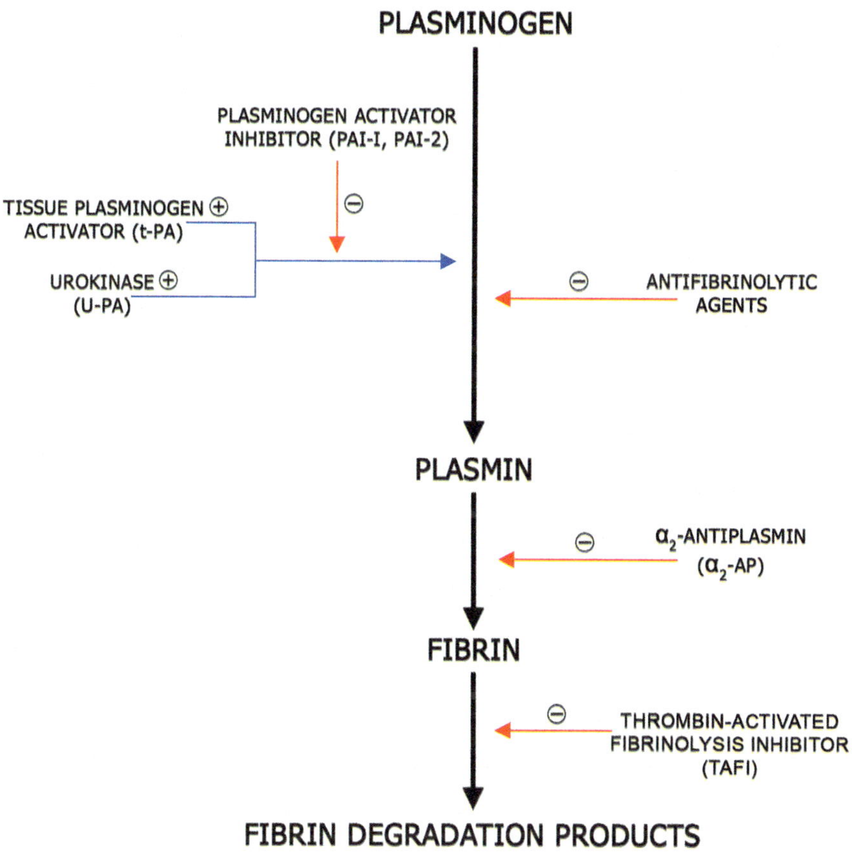

Fig. 2.6 Fibrinolysis

The determination of D-dimer levels is used in the diagnosis of venous thromboembolism. The activation of plasminogen into plasmin under the action of tPA occurs only in the blood clot. It has no effect on systemic fibrinolysis. Free plasmin in circulation is rapidly inactivated being degraded by antiplasmin factors, such as α-2-antiplasmin. In addition to tPa, a strong plasminogen activator is urokinase (uPa). Activated protein C stimulates fibrinolysis by opposing the action of plasminogen activator inhibitors [1, 5, 7, 11].

Contrary to these activators, there are natural inhibitors of fibrinolysis such as plasminogen activator inhibitors (PAI-1 and PAI-2), thrombin-activated fibrinolysis inhibitor (TAFI), and α_2-antiplasmin [5–7, 11].

It is important to note that plasminogen and plasminogen activators are naturally present in saliva and gingival sulcus fluid [14–16]. The fibrinolytic activity of saliva is a leading cause of dry socket and can also contribute to postoperative bleeding in individuals with bleeding disorders, especially those with hemophilia. Therefore, using antifibrinolytics in persons with hemophilia is particularly helpful in preventing postextraction bleeding [17].

References

1. Hall JE, Hall ME. Hemostasis and blood coagulation. In: Hall JE, Hall ME, editors. Guyton and Hall textbook of medical physiology. 14th ed. Philadelphia: Elsevier; 2021. p. 477–88.
2. Kuang T, Szumita RP. Local tissues in hemostasis and platelet review. In: Szumita RP, Szumita PM, editors. Hemostasis in dentistry. Springer eBook; 2018. p. 3–12.
3. Krüger-Genge A, Blocki A, Franke RP, Jung F. Vascular endothelial cell biology: an update. Int J Mol Sci. 2019;20(18):4411.
4. Konkle BA. Disorders of platelets and vessel wall. In section: Disorders of hemostasis. In: Harrison's principles of internal medicine. 20th ed. McGraw-Hill Education eBook; 2018. p. 822–30.
5. Scully C. Haemathology. In: Scully's medical problems in dentistry. 7th ed. Churchill Livingstone: Elsevier; 2014. p. 212–75.
6. Little JW, Miller CS, Rhodus NL. Acquired bleeding and hypercoagulable disorders. In: Little and Falace's dental management of the medically compromised patient. 9th ed. St. Louis: Elsevier; 2018. p. 428–56.
7. Konkle BA. Bleeding and thrombosis. In section: Hematologic alterations. In: Harrison's principles of internal medicine. 20th ed. McGraw-Hill Education eBook; 2018. p. 404–11.
8. Israels S, Schwetz N, Boyar R, McNicol A. Bleeding disorders: characterization, dental considerations and management. J Can Dent Assoc. 2006;72(9):827.
9. Lowe GD. Common risk factors for both arterial and venous thrombosis. Br J Haematol. 2008;140(5):488–95.
10. Previtali E, Bucciarelli P, Passamonti SM, Martinelli I. Risk factors for venous and arterial thrombosis. Blood Transfus. 2011;9(2):120–38.
11. Szumita RP. Coagulation enzymes review and review of hemostasis: putting it all together. In: Szumita RP, Szumita PM, editors. Hemostasis in dentistry. Springer eBook; 2018. p. 14–23.
12. Hoffman M, Monroe DM. Coagulation 2006: a modern view of hemostasis. Hematol Oncol Clin North Am. 2007;21(1):1–11.
13. Romney G, Glick M. An updated concept of coagulation with clinical implications. J Am Dent Assoc. 2009;140(5):567–74.
14. Sindet-Pedersen S, Gram J, Jespersen J. Characterization of plasminogen activators in unstimulated and stimulated human whole saliva. J Dent Res. 1987;66:1199–203.

15. Gersel-Pedersen N. Fibrinolytic activity of blood and saliva before and after oral surgery. Int J Oral Surg. 1981;10(Suppl 1):114–21.
16. Majerus P, Dalcette B, Hermans M, Pourtois M, Capel P. Variations in fibrinolytic activity of human whole saliva. Eur J Oral Sci. 1996;104:341–5.
17. Srivastava A, Santagostino E, Dougall A, Kitchen S, Sutherland M, Pipe SW, Carcao M, Mahlangu J, Ragni MV, Windyga J, Llinás A, Goddard NJ, Mohan R, Poonnoose PM, Feldman BM, Lewis SZ, van den Berg HM, Pierce GF, WFH Guidelines for the Management of Hemophilia panelists and co-authors. WFH Guidelines for the Management of Hemophilia, 3rd edition. Haemophilia. 2020;Suppl 6:1–158. Erratum in: Haemophilia 2021;27(4):699.

Part III

Hemostasis Screening Tests

Basic Laboratory Evaluation of Hemostasis

3

Branislav V. Bajkin and Ivana Urosevic

Bleeding disorders can be classified as vascular disorders, quantitative and qualitative platelet disorders, coagulation factor deficiencies, and fibrinolytic disorders. In addition to medical history, family history, and physical examination, the laboratory testing is essential for the diagnosis of hemostatic disorders. Laboratory testing can indicate the level at which the hemostatic function is impaired. It is important to emphasize that the laboratory assessment of hemostatic function begins with a complete blood count (CBC).

3.1 Laboratory Assessment of Primary Hemostasis

Bleeding time (BT) is an in vivo test that refers to assessment of platelet function in hemostatic plug formation. It is defined as the time needed for bleeding to stop after a standardized incision in the skin. BT is used to evaluate platelet function. The BT normal range is between 1 and 6 min [1]. Prolonged BT is seen in platelet function and/or number disorders and certain blood vessel disorders. BT is not a useful predictor of postoperative bleeding risk and should not be used for this purpose [2, 3].

Platelet count and platelet function assays are necessary for the diagnosis of quantitative and qualitative platelet disorders. Normal platelet count in the blood is $150–450 \times 10^9$/L. A decreased platelet count (thrombocytopenia) may be indicative of several diseases and conditions. There are several methods for assessing platelet function. The most used tests are light transmission platelet aggregometry, whole

B. V. Bajkin (✉)
University of Novi Sad, Faculty of Medicine, Dentistry Clinic of Vojvodina, Novi Sad, Serbia
e-mail: branislav.bajkin@mf.uns.ac.rs

I. Urosevic
University of Novi Sad, Faculty of Medicine, University Clinical Center of Vojvodina, Clinic of Hematology, Novi Sad, Serbia

B. V. Bajkin (ed.), *Bleeding Disorders and Dentistry*,
https://doi.org/10.1007/978-3-032-26713-9_3

blood aggregometry, platelet function analyser-100 (PFA-100), thrombelastography, and flow cytometry (FC) [2, 4–6]. These tests are considered more sensitive and specific for diagnosing platelet function disorders and VWD than BT. However, many of these tests are not used in everyday routine practice, and they are of little value for use in dentistry [3].

3.2 Laboratory Assessment of Coagulation

There are numerous tests used to assess the intrinsic, extrinsic, and common pathways of coagulation (Table 3.1). Prothrombin time (PT) and activated partial thromboplastin time (aPTT) are the two most commonly used in vitro tests to assess the function of coagulation system.

PT is the screening test for the extrinsic and common coagulation pathways. It is helpful in detecting deficiencies of FVII, FII, FV, FX, and fibrinogen. Normal PT values range from 11 to 15 s. PT is commonly reported as an INR (*International Normalized Ratio*), especially in patients taking vitamin K antagonists (VKAs). VKAs inhibit the synthesis of active vitamin K-dependent factors (FII, FVII, FIX, and FX). INR is used to standardize the PT test and represents the ratio of the patient's PT to the mean normal PT, corrected for the sensitivity of the thromboplastin used as a reagent. A normal INR value is 0.9–1.3. PT/INR is used to monitor oral anticoagulant therapy. It is an appropriate tool for predicting the risk of bleeding in patients taking VKAs, but in patients with liver disease, it only partially reflects the bleeding risk because of the complex disorder of hemostasis [1, 2, 4, 7].

aPTT is the screening test for the intrinsic (FVIII, FIX, FXI, FXII, prekallikrein, HMWK) and common coagulation pathway (FV, FX, prothrombin, and fibrinogen) [1, 4]. Normal aPTT values range from 25 to 35 s [3, 7]. The aPTT is prolonged in

Table 3.1 Coagulation tests in hemostatic disorders and in patients taking oral anticoagulant therapy[a]

	PT (INR)	aPTT	TT	Fibrinogen
Hemophilia A and B	Normal	↑	Normal	Normal
VWD	Normal	Normal or ↑	Normal	Normal
Advanced liver disease	↑	↑	Normal or ↑	Normal or ↓
VKA therapy	↑	Normal	Normal	Normal
DOAC				
Dabigatran	Normal or ↑	↑	↑	Normal
FXa inhibitors	Normal or ↑	Normal or ↑	Normal	Normal
DIC	↑	↑	↑	↓

PT prothrombin time, *INR* International Normalized Ratio, *aPTT* activated partial thromboplastin time, *TT* thrombin time, *VWD* von Willebrand disease, *VKA* vitamin K antagonists, *DOAC* direct oral anticoagulants, *DIC* disseminated intravascular coagulation, *FXa inhibitors* rivaroxaban, apixaban, edoxaban

[a]The table requires careful interpretation, considering that the severity of the disease may affect the results of an individual test. For example, depending on the degree of liver insufficiency, PT and aPTT tests may range from normal to significantly prolonged values

patients on heparin therapy and in persons with hemophilia A and B, VWD, and liver disease [4, 7].

Thrombin time (TT) is performed by adding thrombin to the patient's plasma, and it reflects the conversion of fibrinogen to fibrin. It is used to detect quantitative and qualitative deficiencies of fibrinogen [4]. Normal TT values range from 9 to 13 s, while values from 16 to 18 s are prolonged or abnormal [3]. Although TT is not one of the basic screening tests, it is widely used in laboratory evaluation of coagulation disorders. It can be used to measure the anticoagulant effect of dabigatran, direct thrombin inhibitor. Direct oral anticoagulants (DOACs) usually do not require routine monitoring of the anticoagulant effect. If necessary, anti-FXa assay can be used for assessing anticoagulant effect of direct FXa inhibitors.

Deficiency of FXIII, α_2-plasmin inhibitor deficiency, and plasminogen activator inhibitor-1 (PAI-1) deficiency are coagulation and fibrinolytic disorders that do not affect PT, aPTT, and TT [3].

The activated coagulation time is not widely available, and it is not the basic screening test in laboratory evaluation of coagulation disorders.

The evaluation of FVIII and FIX levels should be performed in persons with hemophilia A and hemophilia B, respectively. VWF antigen, VWF activity, and FVIII activity are screening tests for VWD. The evaluation of other factor levels, such as FVII, FXI, and FXII, is required to confirm the deficiency of these factors.

3.3 Fibrinolytic Activity Assessment

Determination of fibrinogen and fibrin degradation products (D-dimers) in plasma is most used for fibrinolysis assessment. Shortened euglobulin clot lysis time is detected in patients with high circulating plasminogen activator levels, in patients with PAI-1 deficiency, and in those with acquired hyperfibrinolysis [4].

References

1. Hall JE, Hall ME. Hemostasis and blood coagulation. In: Hall JE, Hall ME, editors. Guyton and Hall textbook of medical physiology. 14th ed. Philadelphia: Elsevier; 2021. p. 477–88.
2. Konkle BA. Bleeding and thrombosis. In section: Hematologic alterations. In: Harrison's principles of internal medicine. 20th ed. McGraw-Hill Education eBook; 2018. p. 404–11.
3. Little JW, Miller CS, Rhodus NL. Acquired bleeding and hypercoagulable disorders. In: Little and Falace's dental management of the medically compromised patient. 9th ed. St. Louis: Elsevier; 2018. p. 428–56.
4. Hayward CPM. How I investigate for bleeding disorders. Int J Lab Hematol. 2018;40(Suppl 1):6–14.
5. Rand ML, Reddy EC, Israels SJ. Laboratory diagnosis of inherited platelet function disorders. Transfus Apher Sci. 2018;57(4):485–93.
6. Israels SJ. Laboratory testing for platelet function disorders. Int J Lab Hematol. 2015;37(Suppl 1):18–24.
7. Scully C. Haemathology. In: Scully's medical problems in dentistry. 7th ed. Churchill Livingstone: Elsevier; 2014. p. 212–75.

Part IV

Bleeding Disorders and Dentistry

Classification of Hemostatic Disorders

4

Branislav V. Bajkin and Ivana Urosevic

The function of normal hemostasis is to keep the blood in a liquid state and allow blood flow within blood vessels but also to prevent blood outflow in normal conditions or lead to cessation of bleeding when the vessel is damaged. Hemostatic disorders can be classified into two major groups: hemorrhagic syndromes and thrombotic disorders.

Dental management of patients with hemorrhagic syndromes is of great importance; therefore, these disorders are in the focus of this book. According to the cause of the disorder, bleeding disorders can be classified into vasculopathies, disorders of platelet function or number, and coagulopathies. Hemorrhagic syndromes can also be divided into congenital and acquired disorders (Table 4.1).

Anticoagulant and antiplatelet drugs are used in prevention and treatment of thrombosis and thromboembolic complications. Thrombotic disorders are mostly presented in the book from the perspective of bleeding tendency associated with the use of antithrombotic drugs.

Given the large number of hemorrhagic disorders and their complexity, the book focuses on the most important diseases in terms of dental treatment. Etiopathogenesis, clinical findings, therapy, and current dental recommendation for treatment of patients with bleeding disorders are presented in the book.

B. V. Bajkin (✉)
University of Novi Sad, Faculty of Medicine, Dentistry Clinic of Vojvodina, Novi Sad, Serbia
e-mail: branislav.bajkin@mf.uns.ac.rs

I. Urosevic
University of Novi Sad, Faculty of Medicine, University Clinical Center of Vojvodina,
Clinic of Hematology, Novi Sad, Serbia

B. V. Bajkin (ed.), *Bleeding Disorders and Dentistry*,
https://doi.org/10.1007/978-3-032-26713-9_4

Table 4.1 Acquired and congenital bleeding disorders

	Acquired	Congenital
Disorders of the vessel wall (vascular purpura)	Scurvy (vitamin C deficiency) Metabolic disorders Infections Allergy Henoch-Schönlein purpura	Hereditary hemorrhagic telangiectasia (Osler-Weber-Rendu-disease)
Platelet function disorders	Antiplatelet drugs High-dose penicillins Uremia Autoimmune disease Hematologic disorders	Glanzmann thrombasthenia Bernard-Soulier disease[a] Storage pool deficiency Secretion platelet defects Others von Willebrand disease[b]
Platelet number disorders (thrombocytopenic purpura)	Idiopathic Bacterial and viral infections Drug-induced thrombocytopenia Systemic autoimmune diseases (systemic lupus erythematosus, rheumatoid arthritis, antiphospholipid syndrome, and others) Splenomegaly Mechanical prosthetic heart valves Malignant diseases (leukemia, myeloma multiplex, bone metastases, and others) Radiation Chemical agents Alcohol Disseminated intravascular coagulation	May-Hegglin anomaly Sebastian syndrome Fechtner syndrome Epstein syndrome Others
Coagulation disorders	Liver disease Vitamin K deficiency Anticoagulation drugs (heparin, vitamin K antagonists, direct oral anticoagulants) Disseminated intravascular coagulation	Hemophilia A Hemophilia B FXI deficiency Rare coagulopathies

[a]Also classified as thrombocytopenic disorder
[b]Due to FVIII deficiency in severe forms, there is also defect in coagulation

Disorders of the Blood Vessel Wall

5

Branislav V. Bajkin and Ivana Urosevic

Vascular bleeding disorders are referred to as vascular purpuras and can be inherited and acquired. The most common inherited disorder of the vessel wall is hereditary hemorrhagic telangiectasia (HHT) or Osler-Weber-Rendu disease (OWRD). Easy bruising and frequent bleeding can be clinical manifestations of inherited connective tissue diseases, such as Marfan syndrome and Ehlers-Danlos syndrome. Blood vessels can also be affected by numerous metabolic and inflammatory diseases, such as vasculitis [1].

5.1 Hereditary Hemorrhagic Telangiectasia (Osler-Weber-Rendu Disease)

HHT is an autosomal dominant inherited disease in which the elastic and muscle components of blood vessels are primarily affected, resulting in telangiectasia or vascular malformations. The disease may present in multiple clinical forms, most commonly as hereditary hemorrhagic telangiectasia 1 and 2 (HHT1 and HHT2). The cause of HHT1 is a mutation in the endoglin gene located on chromosome 9. Endoglin mutation leads to ineffective binding of transforming grow factor beta (TGF_{β}) to receptors on endothelium and smooth muscles. TGF_{β} is involved in triggering signaling mechanisms required for vascular development. This form of the disease is usually more severe and often includes the presence of arteriovenous malformations in the lungs and brain. HHT2 is the result of a mutation in the gene for activin receptor-like-kinase-1 (ALK-1) located on chromosome 12. ALK-1 is a

B. V. Bajkin (✉)
University of Novi Sad, Faculty of Medicine, Dentistry Clinic of Vojvodina, Novi Sad, Serbia
e-mail: branislav.bajkin@mf.uns.ac.rs

I. Urosevic
University of Novi Sad, Faculty of Medicine, University Clinical Center of Vojvodina, Clinic of Hematology, Novi Sad, Serbia

B. V. Bajkin (ed.), *Bleeding Disorders and Dentistry*,
https://doi.org/10.1007/978-3-032-26713-9_5

protein that forms a complex with endoglin and TGF_β on the surface of endothelial cells. Both forms of the disease, HHT1 and HHT2, share the same underlying mechanism, disruption of the signaling cascade on endothelial cells that involves TGF_β and vascular endothelial growth factor (VEGF) resulting in the disorder in angiogenesis, tendency toward their easy injury, and the formation of arteriovenous malformations. HHT2 is a less severe form, which subsequently manifests later in life [2–5].

The prevalence of HHT in the general population is about 1:5000 [4, 6]. The disease can be heterogenous regarding the clinical manifestations. It can be asymptomatic for many years or exhibit varying degree of severity from mild forms with mucocutaneous telangiectasia to serious forms with multiple arteriovenous malformations in numerous organs. Clinical symptoms usually develop over time, with recurrent epistaxis being the leading symptom, present in more than 95% of patients with OWRD [1, 6]. Vascular abnormalities can be seen in various regions and involve different organs: skin, nasal mucosa, lungs, brain, eye, liver, and gastrointestinal tract including the oral cavity [4, 7]. Skin lesions are most often seen on the fingers, face, extremities, and trunk [1, 6]. Bleeding from the gastrointestinal tract may manifest as acute gastrointestinal bleeding but may remain clinically unapparent and cause anemia. The involvement of central nervous system may have various clinical manifestations such as migraines, epilepsy, ischemic cerebrovascular attacks, brain abscess, and intracranial hemorrhages. Clinical symptoms of pulmonary arteriovenous malformations are usually absent until complications occur. The complications include massive hemoptysis and spontaneous hemothorax [6].

The disease is most often diagnosed by rhinoscopy in case of recurrent epistaxis, gastrointestinal tract endoscopy, or dental examination when telangiectatic changes are present in oral cavity. Appropriate radiographic imaging is used for the diagnosis of vascular malformations in internal organs. Along with thorough physical examination and radiographic imaging, a positive family history and genetic testing may aid in reaching a definitive diagnosis. Diagnosis of the disease is based on Curaçao criteria: (1) epistaxis, (2) cutaneous or mucosal telangiectasia, (3) visceral arteriovenous malformations, and (4) positive family history in the first-degree relatives. The disease is suspected or considered likely if two of these criteria are met, and a definitive diagnosis made if three out of four criteria are fulfilled [2]. Genetic testing helps in the diagnosis especially in asymptomatic individuals with a positive family history [4, 6].

Management of HHT is individual and depends on the location of vascular malformations and clinical manifestations of the disease. The therapy includes moisturizing of the nasal mucosa to prevent epistaxis, iron supplementation (in case of anemia) due to bleeding from the gastrointestinal tract, the use of antifibrinolytics, intravenous administration of bevacizumab (anti-VEGF monoclonal antibody), or other systemic antiangiogenic therapy. Surgical treatment and lasers or electrocautery are used to achieve hemostasis and remove minor telangiectatic changes. The application of local hemostatic agents and other measures are taken to stop bleeding from accessible sites such as nosebleeds or oral bleeding [4, 6–8].

5.2 Metabolic and Inflammatory Diseases of Blood Vessels

Blood vessels can be affected by numerous metabolic and inflammatory diseases and conditions such as those in acute febrile conditions related to viral infections, Rocky-Mountain spotted fever, Waldenström's macroglobulinemia, multiple myeloma, and cryoglobulinemia [1]. The underlying mechanisms of these diseases involve either direct endothelial damage by an infectious agent or immune-mediated damage of blood vessel wall. Less common forms of vascular purpura include mixed cryoglobulinemia, which can be an extrahepatic manifestation of hepatitis C infection, and purpura as a cutaneous manifestation of systemic amyloidosis. In patients with Cushing's syndrome or those on long-term corticosteroid therapy, there is a bleeding tendency due to atrophy of the supporting connective tissue around blood vessels. Similar changes can be seen in the elderly following minor trauma, presenting as superficial bleeding within the skin especially in areas that have often been exposed to the sun (senile purpura) [1].

Scurvy is a manifestation of vitamin C deficiency, resulting in impaired collagen synthesis. Vitamin C is essential for the synthesis of hydroxyproline as a component of collagen. Commonly, scurvy is a consequence of malnutrition, specifically of a poor or unbalanced diet, and excessive alcohol consumption. Clinical signs of the disease include slow wound healing, gingival bleeding, painless perifollicular hemorrhages, and ecchymoses. In addition to gum bleeding, tooth decay is frequently observed. The diagnosis is clinically determined based on malnutrition and bleeding manifestations, while hemostatic screening tests are normal. The therapeutic use of vitamin C leads to a rapid resolution of symptoms [1, 9].

Henoch-Schönlein purpura (HSP) or anaphylactoid purpura or IgA vasculitis is a systemic vasculitis that affects small blood vessels primarily in the skin, joints, mucosa of the gastrointestinal tract, and kidneys and, less frequently, the lungs and central nervous system. Pathogenic mechanism of this disease is the formation of antigen/antibody complex, primarily IgA class antibodies, that leads to activation of complement components and accumulation of neutrophils, resulting in inflammation and increased permeability of venules, capillaries, and smaller arterioles and localized bleeding. The etiology of the disease is unknown, but it is believed that immune, genetic, and environmental factors play a major role in its development [10].

The disease typically manifests in childhood and adolescence and less frequently in adulthood. HSP is the most common vasculitis in childhood, and estimated prevalence is 10–20 cases per 100,000 school children annually [10]. The highest incidence is observed in children aged 2–10 years, with a peak onset around 6 years of age. The disease is more common in boys and during winter months. The onset of purpura is usually preceded by an upper respiratory tract infection—streptococcal pharyngitis. HSP is also associated with other infections, certain vaccines, and food and drug allergies. The presence of IgA deposits is most associated with mucosal infection in the mouth, ear, nose, and throat.

The major clinical features of HSP include palpable purpuric skin rash on the extensor surfaces of the legs and arms, arthritis or arthralgia of large joints, diffuse abdominal pain in the form of colic which may be accompanied by vomiting and bleeding from gastrointestinal tract, and hematuria/proteinuria due to proliferative glomerulonephritis [1, 10]. Some of the symptoms may be absent from the clinical presentation. The skin manifestations are in the form of palpable red-purple purpura or petechial rash usually symmetrically distributed over areas exposed to pressure or in areas most affected by gravity. Skin lesions can be confluent, non-blanching on palpation, non-pruritic, and non-painful. The severity of the clinical presentation primarily depends on the extent of renal involvement. HSP nephritis can be seen in about 40% of children with HSP [10]. In certain cases, the disease may progress to end-stage renal disease; therefore, HSP patients require long-term monitoring of kidney function following the diagnosis.

The diagnosis is based on the clinical manifestations of purpura most often presented on the lower extremities and pain in the ankle and knee joints among patients of younger ages. Medical history often reveals recent upper respiratory tract infection. Laboratory tests show elevated IgA levels, and in the case of renal involvement, hematuria and proteinuria are typically present. Screening tests for hemostasis including platelet counts are normal, which clearly distinguishes HSP from immune thrombocytopenic purpura (ITP). No single symptom or individual laboratory test is sufficient for establishing the diagnosis. The diagnosis is confirmed by the presence of palpable purpura along with at least one of the following four criteria: acute diffuse abdominal pain, arthritis or arthralgia, renal involvement (hematuria and/or proteinuria), or predominant IgA deposits in biopsy specimens, related to leucocytoclastic vasculitis or proliferative glomerulonephritis [11].

The therapy is mainly symptomatic. In mild forms of the disease, spontaneous recovery usually occurs within 4 weeks without sequelae. The main prognostic factor of the disease is kidney involvement, i.e., the presence of hematuria and/or proteinuria. In case of systemic manifestations, particularly the development of glomerulonephritis, treatment includes the use of corticosteroids, which provide symptomatic relief but do not alter the course of the disease [1]. In severe forms, immunosuppressive agents such as cyclophosphamide, cyclosporine, and azathioprine can be used; however, their use is controversial. In a certain number of cases, kidney impairment may remain as a lasting consequence and may reoccur following clinical improvement healing [10].

References

1. Konkle BA. Disorders of platelets and vessel wall. In section: Disorders of hemostasis. In: Harrison's principles of internal medicine. 20th ed. McGraw-Hill Education eBook; 2018. p. 822–30.
2. Shovlin CL, Guttmacher AE, Buscarini E, Faughnan ME, Hyland RH, Westermann CJ, Kjeldsen AD, Plauchu H. Diagnostic criteria for hereditary hemorrhagic telangiectasia (Rendu-Osler-Weber syndrome). Am J Med Genet. 2000;91(1):66–7.
3. Shovlin CL. Hereditary haemorrhagic telangiectasia: pathophysiology, diagnosis and treatment. Blood Rev. 2010;24(6):203–19.

4. Faughnan ME, Mager JJ, Hetts SW, Palda VA, Lang-Robertson K, Buscarini E, Deslandres E, Kasthuri RS, Lausman A, Poetker D, Ratjen F, Chesnutt MS, Clancy M, Whitehead KJ, Al-Samkari H, Chakinala M, Conrad M, Cortes D, Crocione C, Darling J, de Gussem E, Derksen C, Dupuis-Girod S, Foy P, Geisthoff U, Gossage JR, Hammill A, Heimdal K, Henderson K, Iyer VN, Kjeldsen AD, Komiyama M, Korenblatt K, McDonald J, McMahon J, McWilliams J, Meek ME, Mei-Zahav M, Olitsky S, Palmer S, Pantalone R, Piccirillo JF, Plahn B, Porteous MEM, Post MC, Radovanovic I, Rochon PJ, Rodriguez-Lopez J, Sabba C, Serra M, Shovlin C, Sprecher D, White AJ, Winship I, Zarrabeitia R. Second international guidelines for the diagnosis and management of hereditary hemorrhagic telangiectasia. Ann Intern Med. 2020;173(12):989–1001.
5. da Silva Santos PS, Fernandes KS, Magalhães MH. Osler-Weber-Rendu syndrome--dental implications. J Can Dent Assoc. 2009;75(7):527–30.
6. Faughnan ME, Palda VA, Garcia-Tsao G, Geisthoff UW, McDonald J, Proctor DD, Spears J, Brown DH, Buscarini E, Chesnutt MS, Cottin V, Ganguly A, Gossage JR, Guttmacher AE, Hyland RH, Kennedy SJ, Korzenik J, Mager JJ, Ozanne AP, Piccirillo JF, Picus D, Plauchu H, Porteous ME, Pyeritz RE, Ross DA, Sabba C, Swanson K, Terry P, Wallace MC, Westermann CJ, White RI, Young LH, Zarrabeitia R, HHT Foundation International – Guidelines Working Group. International guidelines for the diagnosis and management of hereditary haemorrhagic telangiectasia. J Med Genet. 2011;48(2):73–87.
7. Little JW, Miller CS, Rhodus NL. Congenital bleeding and hypercoagulable disorders. In: Little and Falace's dental management of the medically compromised patient. 9th ed. St. Louis: Elsevier; 2018. p. 457–79.
8. Al-Samkari H. Hereditary hemorrhagic telangiectasia: systemic therapies, guidelines, and an evolving standard of care. Blood. 2021;137(7):888–95.
9. Hall JE, Hall ME. Dietary balances; regulation of feeding; obesity and starvation; vitamins and minerals. In: Hall JE, Hall ME, editors. Guyton and Hall textbook of medical physiology. 14th ed. Philadelphia: Elsevier; 2021. p. 877–92.
10. Leung AKC, Barankin B, Leong KF. Henoch-Schönlein purpura in children: an updated review. Curr Pediatr Rev. 2020;16(4):265–76.
11. Ozen S, Pistorio A, Iusan SM, Bakkaloglu A, Herlin T, Brik R, Buoncompagni A, Lazar C, Bilge I, Uziel Y, Rigante D, Cantarini L, Hilario MO, Silva CA, Alegria M, Norambuena X, Belot A, Berkun Y, Estrella AI, Olivieri AN, Alpigiani MG, Rumba I, Sztajnbok F, Tambic-Bukovac L, Breda L, Al-Mayouf S, Mihaylova D, Chasnyk V, Sengler C, Klein-Gitelman M, Djeddi D, Nuno L, Pruunsild C, Brunner J, Kondi A, Pagava K, Pederzoli S, Martini A, Ruperto N, Paediatric Rheumatology International Trials Organisation (PRINTO). EULAR/PRINTO/PRES criteria for Henoch-Schönlein purpura, childhood polyarteritis nodosa, childhood Wegener granulomatosis and childhood Takayasu arteritis: Ankara 2008. Part II: Final classification criteria. Ann Rheum Dis. 2010;69(5):798–806.

6 Dental Considerations in Patients with Vascular Bleeding Disorders

Branislav V. Bajkin and Alison Dougall

Box 6.1 Dental Considerations in Patients with Vascular Bleeding Disorders

1. *Hereditary* disorders (Osler-Weber-Rendu disease, OWRD)
2. *Metabolic and inflammatory disorders* (infections, immune-mediated vasculitis, scurvy, Henoch-Schönlein purpura)

Dental Considerations

- Oral manifestations of vascular bleeding disorders
- Importance of maintaining oral hygiene
- Dental treatment may require modification regarding the severity of the disease
- Consultation with patient's physician
- Laboratory tests usually not necessary for invasive dental procedure
- Consider antibiotic prophylaxis in patients with OWRD and arteriovenous malformation
- Use of local anesthesia with vasoconstrictor
- Minimally traumatic surgical technique
- Use of local hemostatic agents and measures to control oral bleeding
- Provide a patient with postoperative instructions (avoid aspirin and other NSAIDs, soft and cold diet, phone number in case of an emergency) and regular follow-up

NSAIDs nonsteroidal anti-inflammatory drugs

B. V. Bajkin (✉)
University of Novi Sad, Faculty of Medicine, Dentistry Clinic of Vojvodina, Novi Sad, Serbia
e-mail: branislav.bajkin@mf.uns.ac.rs

A. Dougall
School of Dental Science, Trinity College Dublin, Dublin Dental University Hospital, Dublin, Ireland

B. V. Bajkin (ed.), *Bleeding Disorders and Dentistry*,
https://doi.org/10.1007/978-3-032-26713-9_6

Oral manifestations and dental managing of patients with the most common vasculopathies HHT and HSP will be presented in this chapter.

6.1 Dental Management of Patients with Hereditary Hemorrhagic Telangiectasia

Expertise of dentists requires the knowledge about the manifestations of HHT, considering that lesions in the oral cavity are sometimes the first sign of the disease. The disease typically presents clinically in the second and third decade of life. Telangiectatic changes in the oral cavity are most often registered on the tongue and vermilion of the lip, gingiva, mucosa of the mouth floor, and palate (Fig. 6.1).

Dental treatment may sometimes need to be modified depending on the severity of clinical manifestations and potential involvement of various organs and systems. Patients with arteriovenous malformations in the lungs should not be placed supine during dental treatment as this can cause hypoxia. The presence of pulmonary arteriovenous malformations and vascular lesions in the brain may increase the risk of developing brain abscess, being one of the most serious complications in patients with HHT with high rate of mortality. For this reason, some authors have suggested antibiotic prophylaxis for any invasive dental procedure [1, 2]. However, antibiotic prophylaxis in HHT patients remains highly controversial [3]. Some authors stated that due to the lack of solid evidence, there are no clear benefits of using antibiotics in such cases [4]. In support to this is the current prevailing view that repeated bacteremia caused by poor oral hygiene is considered a more common cause of distant infections than the risk posed by a single dental procedure. For this reason, it is essential to emphasize to patients the importance of maintaining proper oral hygiene.

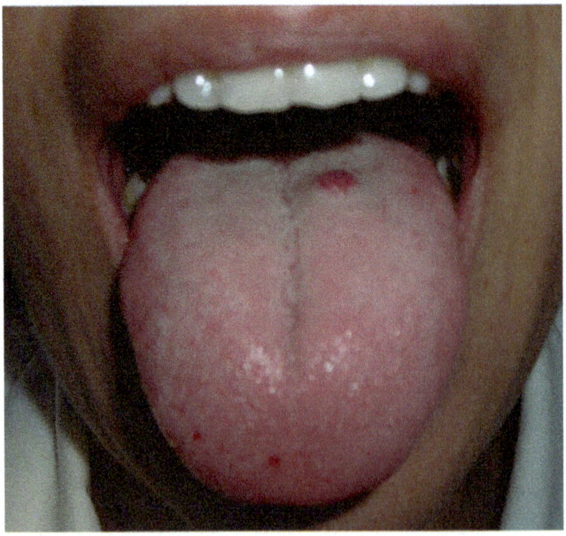

Fig. 6.1 Oral manifestations of hereditary hemorrhagic telangiectasia

In severe forms of HHT, the degree of anemia and the risks associated with more extensive oral or maxillofacial surgical procedures need to be assessed. Although cases of life-threatening bleeding from the oral cavity in patients with HHT have been reported [3], bleeding from oral cavity lesions is usually mild and can be easily controlled by local hemostatic agents and measures [5].

6.2 Dental Management of Patients with Henoch-Schönlein Purpura

It is frequently reported in the literature that there is an association between poor oral health and chronic inflammation in the oral cavity on one hand and the development and severity of clinical manifestation of HSP on the other [6–9]. Data also suggest that infections in the oral cavity and certain dental procedures such as tooth extraction, endodontic treatment, or periodontal procedures may serve as a trigger for the development of HSP [6, 10], whereas removal of dental foci can lead to faster recovery from this disease [11, 12]. On the other hand, a high prevalence and possibly a greater susceptibility to the development of oral diseases such as tooth decay and apical periodontitis have been observed in children with HSP [6]. It is widely accepted that a local infection within the oral cavity commonly found at the apices of non-vital teeth or because of periodontal diseases may lead to systemic infection. A vast number of aerobic and anaerobic bacteria constitute the microbiome of the oral cavity and carious lesions (50–100 billion bacteria representing 500–700 different species). Toxins and degradation products of these bacteria stimulate the production of inflammatory cytokines by cellular elements in periapical lesions, which may trigger a systemic immune response. Additionally, bacteria from a localized focus can enter the bloodstream, leading to bacteremia and their dissemination, which may result in endothelial damage and the activation of immune processes. The results of recent studies utilizing next-generation sequencing support a potential association and possible influence of oral cavity bacteria in the development of HSP. A difference has been identified in the oral microbiome between children with HSP and healthy controls. An increased bacterial load as well as greater microbial diversity has been observed in children with HSP [13].

The severity of the clinical presentation and the outcome of the disease depend on the renal involvement. Any focal infection, including those in the oral cavity, presents a risk factor for further kidney damage and should be identified and treated promptly. In consultation with the attending physician, the need for antibiotic prophylaxis should be considered before an invasive dental procedure in patients with HSP and renal impairment.

Dental treatment in children with HSP must focus on the preservation and maintenance of oral health including the restoration of all teeth with carious lesions, management of teeth with pulpitis and periapical lesions, as well as the treatment of gum diseases. It is of utmost importance to implement dental measures and procedures for the prevention of oral and dental diseases such as motivation and training on proper oral hygiene maintenance, dietary recommendations, regular dental visits, local fluoride application, and pit and fissure sealing.

References

1. da Silva Santos PS, Fernandes KS, Magalhães MH. Osler-Weber-Rendu syndrome—dental implications. J Can Dent Assoc. 2009;75(7):527–30.
2. Corre P, Perret C, Isidor B, Khonsari RH. A brain abscess following dental extractions in a patient with hereditary hemorrhagic telangiectasia. Br J Oral Maxillofac Surg. 2011;49(5):e9–11.
3. Ahamed SK, Al-Thobaiti Y. Life-threatening oral bleed—a rare presentation of hereditary hemorrhagic telangiectasia. J Oral Maxillofac Surg. 2015;73(8):1465.e1–5.
4. te Veldhuis EC, te Veldhuis AH, van Dijk FS, Kwee ML, van Hagen JM, Baart JA, van der Waal I. Rendu-Osler-Weber disease: update of medical and dental considerations. Oral Surg Oral Med Oral Pathol Oral Radiol Endod. 2008;105(2):e38–41.
5. Hopp RN, de Siqueira DC, Sena-Filho M, Jorge J. Oral vascular malformation in a patient with hereditary hemorrhagic telangiectasia: a case report. Spec Care Dentist. 2013;33(3):150–3.
6. Echavarría-García AC, Pozos-Guillén A, Tejeda-Nava F, Flores Arriaga JC, Garrocho-Rangel A. Oral management of children with Henoch-Schönlein Purpura and associated glomerulonephritis: a scoping review. Eur J Paediatr Dent. 2018;19(2):134–8.
7. Enzenauer RJ, Sutley SH, Enzenauer RW. Recurrent Henoch-Schonlein purpura presenting as gingival petechiae and mandibular pain. J Oral Maxillofac Surg. 1990;48(6):634–7.
8. Igawa K, Satoh T, Yokozeki H. Possible association of Henoch-Schonlein purpura in adults with odontogenic focal infection. Int J Dermatol. 2011;50(3):277–9.
9. Ghrahani R, Ledika A, Sapartini G, Setiabudiawan B. Age of onset as a risk factor of renal involvement in Henoch-Schönlein purpura. Asia Pacific Assoc Allergy Asthma Clin Imunol. 2014;4:42–7.
10. Tahmassebi JF, Paterson SA. Development of acute Henoch-Schönlein purpura subsequent to endodontic treatment. Int J Paediatr Dent. 2007;17(3):217–22.
11. Abe M, Mori Y, Saijo H, Hoshi K, Ohkubo K, Ono T, Takato T. The efficacy of dental therapy for an adult case of Henoch-Schönlein purpura. Oral Sci Int. 2012;9(2):59–62.
12. Inoue CN, Nagasaka T, Matsutani S, Ishidoya M, Homma R, Chiba Y. Efficacy of early dental and ENT therapy in preventing nephropathy in pediatric Henoch-Schönlein purpura. Clin Rheumatol. 2008;27(12):1489–96.
13. Chen B, Wang J, Wang Y, Zhang J, Zhao C, Shen N, Yang J, Gai Z, Zhang L. Oral microbiota dysbiosis and its association with Henoch-Schönlein Purpura in children. Int Immunopharmacol. 2018;65:295–302.

Disorders of Platelet Number and Function

7

Branislav V. Bajkin and Ivana Urosevic

Platelet disorders may be classified into platelet number disorders (thrombocytopenia or thrombocytosis), platelet function disorders (thrombasthenia), or both platelet count and function disorders. Platelet disorders can be inherited or acquired. Regardless of type of the platelet disorder (qualitative or quantitative), it can be associated with a significant risk of bleeding. Hemorrhages may be spontaneous or induced by some trauma or surgery, including dental procedures.

7.1 Thrombocytopenia

The normal platelet count in the blood ranges from 150 to 400 × 10^9/L, but the number may vary among individuals. Thrombocytopenia refers to a decrease in the platelet count below 150 × 10^9/L, and it is classified depending on the platelet number into mild (100–150 × 10^9/L), moderate (50–99 × 10^9/L), and severe (<50 × 10^9/L) [1, 2]. A platelet count <30 × 10^9/L, particularly <10 × 10^9/L, is associated with a significant risk of spontaneous bleeding, particularly in gastrointestinal and genitourinary tract, and depending on the clinical manifestation may require a transfusion of platelet concentrate [3].

Thrombocytopenia can be either an inherited or acquired disorder, caused by decreased platelet production in the bone marrow, increased sequestration of platelets in the spleen, or their increased breakdown. It can also be a consequence of hemodilution or platelet consumption due to the formation of blood clots [3, 4]. In a majority of cases, a single mechanism leads to thrombocytopenia; however, it may

B. V. Bajkin (✉)
University of Novi Sad, Faculty of Medicine, Dentistry Clinic of Vojvodina, Novi Sad, Serbia
e-mail: branislav.bajkin@mf.uns.ac.rs

I. Urosevic
University of Novi Sad, Faculty of Medicine, University Clinical Center of Vojvodina, Clinic of Hematology, Novi Sad, Serbia

B. V. Bajkin (ed.), *Bleeding Disorders and Dentistry*,
https://doi.org/10.1007/978-3-032-26713-9_7

also be caused by a combination of multiple concurrent mechanisms and contributing factors. Inherited thrombocytopenias are rare diseases, whereas acquired forms may be caused by various factors and mechanisms.

7.1.1 Decreased Platelet Production

A low platelet count due to decreased platelet production may be congenital, but it is far more commonly acquired caused by various factors such as inadequate nutrition or a bone marrow disorder [4].

Congenital thrombocytopenia is a rare disorder, whether it is presented as an isolated condition or part of a syndrome. It can be inherited as autosomal dominant, autosomal recessive, or X-linked disease. Platelet size can be normal, increased, or decreased [4–6]. May-Hegglin anomaly and Sebastian, Epstein, and Fechtner syndrome are autosomal dominant diseases caused by mutations in the MYH9 gene. These diseases have different clinical manifestations and are characterized by thrombocytopenia, large platelets, and inclusions in neutrophils. Congenital amegakaryocytic thrombocytopenia is an autosomal recessive disorder caused by mutation that affects the thrombopoietin receptor. It manifests as severe bleeding shortly after birth. Bernard-Soulier syndrome (BSS) is also an autosomal recessive disease, which, in addition to thrombocytopenia and large platelets, is primarily characterized by functional platelet disorder and will be described in Sect. 7.3. X-linked inherited thrombocytopenias are Wiskott-Aldrich syndrome and thrombocytopenia due to hematopoietic transcription factor GATA-1 mutation [1, 4, 5]. The number of congenital thrombocytopenias is large, and given the low incidence of these conditions, their overall listing exceeds the necessary knowledge in daily dental practice. In most patients with congenital thrombocytopenias, the disease is diagnosed later in life due to mild clinical signs such as mucocutaneous purpura, petechiae, ecchymosis, or mild bleeding following trauma. Family history, along with genetic testing, greatly contributes significantly in the diagnostic process [1, 6].

Acquired thrombocytopenia may result from a deficiency of certain nutrients, in which case other blood cell lineages are usually affected as well and rarely only the thrombocytic lineage. In addition to anemia, deficiencies in iron, vitamin B12 (cobalamin), and vitamin B9 (folic acid) can also be a cause of thrombocytopenia due to decreased megakaryocyte maturation. Excessive alcohol consumption is a common cause of thrombocytopenia. Thrombocytopenia in this case is either caused by alcohol-induced bone marrow suppression (due to the direct effect of alcohol or effect of acetaldehyde, a metabolite of alcohol, on the bone marrow) or by deficiency of folic acid or by splenomegaly and increased platelet sequestration due to terminal liver disease [1, 5, 7]. Decreased platelet production can be a result of bone marrow suppression from an infection (viral infections with human papilloma virus B19, rubella, Epstein-Barr virus, cytomegalovirus, HIV) or suppression caused by drugs, such as chemotherapy agents (see Sect. 7.1.4), or a result of bone marrow infiltration by malignant cells [1, 5, 7]. Bone marrow malignant infiltration does not lead to isolated thrombocytopenia, but rather to pancytopenia. Thrombocytopenia is most commonly caused by massive bone marrow infiltration of hematological tumor cells such as leukemia, multiple myeloma, and lymphoma or bone metastases of solid tumors such as breast, prostate, and lung malignancies. Thrombocytopenia as part of pancytopenia is also seen in myelodysplastic syndromes, which are characterized by ineffective hematopoiesis due to abnormal maturation of bone marrow hematopoietic stem cells.

7.1.2 Increased Platelet Sequestration

It is estimated that about 30% of the total number of platelets are stored in the spleen as an exchangeable pool, which can be released in circulation when needed. The spleen is also a removal site of damaged and old platelets from the circulation. In the setting of hypersplenism, most commonly secondary to liver cirrhosis and portal hypertension, a reduced number of circulating platelets arises due to increased sequestration of platelets within the spleen. Patients with liver disease usually have moderate thrombocytopenia with platelet count from 50 to $100 \times 10^9/L$ [1, 3]. Thrombocytopenia in conjunction with coagulation impairment further compromises hemostatic function in patients with liver disease (see Chap. 14). Splenomegaly accompanied by pancytopenia is seen in myelofibrosis due to the replacement of hematopoietic with fibrous tissue in the bone marrow. Extrahepatic hematopoiesis leads to splenomegaly and consequent thrombocytopenia due to increased platelet sequestration in the spleen [1, 7]. Additionally, splenomegaly can arise as part of the clinical manifestation of various infections, systemic lupus erythematosus (SLE), and inherited lysosomal storage disorders (Gaucher disease, Niemann-Pick disease).

7.1.3 Increased Platelet Degradation

In the setting of accelerated platelet destruction, it is of critical importance to determine whether the process is immune-mediated or not. The most common immune--mediated mechanisms of platelet destruction include immune thrombocytopenic purpura and drug-induced thrombocytopenias. The most frequent thrombocytopenias due to accelerated nonimmune platelet degradation are thrombotic thrombocytopenic purpura, hemolytic-uremic syndrome, heparin-induced thrombocytopenia, and thrombocytopenia as part of disseminated intravascular coagulation.

Immune thrombocytopenia or immune thrombocytopenic purpura (ITP) is a disorder primarily caused by immune-mediated platelet destruction and possibly decreased platelet production in the bone marrow [4]. Antibodies are of the IgG class, and they are most commonly directed against GpIIb/IIIa receptors and less often against GpIb receptors [1, 3]. Antiplatelet antibodies bind to platelets resulting in increased platelet destruction by the reticuloendothelial system. In 80% of patients with ITP, the cause of the disease remains unknown, and it is referred to as idiopathic or primary thrombocytopenia.

Secondary ITP is present in approximately 20% of all cases and occurs as part of another underlying disease, most commonly an autoimmune disorder, such as SLE, antiphospholipid syndrome, rheumatoid arthritis and Sjögren syndrome, and malignant disease or infections, such as HIV and hepatitis C [1, 4]. The disease can also develop during pregnancy. ITP is seen in children and adults but has a different course of the disease. In children, the onset of the disease is usually preceded by one of the common infections at this age, such as varicella zoster, Epstein-Barr, rubella, and others. It has an acute course and a good prognosis and usually resolves spontaneously within a few months [1, 4, 8]. In the adult population, the disease develops gradually and has a chronic course, and remissions are less frequent. ITP is one of the most common forms of thrombocytopenia with an incidence in the adult population of approximately 4:100,000 [1, 8].

Clinical manifestation of ITP depends on the severity of thrombocytopenia. The clinical picture is dominated by mucocutaneous bleeding, most commonly in the oral cavity (wet purpura) (Fig. 1.1a, b), gastrointestinal system or excessive menstrual bleeding in women. In rare cases, bleeding into the central nervous system may occur, posing a life-threatening risk to the patient [4]. Laboratory results show a low platelet count. The platelets can be enlarged but are of normal morphology. In case of more severe bleeding, laboratory findings may indicate anemia. Antibody testing is not routinely performed due to its low sensitivity and specificity. Bone marrow aspiration and biopsy is reserved only for cases of unclear etiology. The final diagnosis is usually made by excluding other conditions that are considered in the differential diagnosis, such as thrombotic thrombocytopenic purpura, liver diseases, aplastic anemia, leukemia, type IIb VWD, drug-induced thrombocytopenia, and myeloproliferative diseases. Diagnostic evaluation should be directed toward confirming secondary ITP, including serological testing for SLE, hepatitis C, or HIV infection.

The therapeutic approach for ITP patients depends on the clinical manifestations of the disease and platelet count. Treatment is usually not necessary in mild cases. In more severe forms and in cases with significant low platelet count, treatment can be aimed at reducing the destruction of antibody-platelet complexes by the reticuloendothelial system, decreasing antibody production, and increasing platelet production [4]. Initial treatment in patients with a severe clinical form involves the administration of corticosteroids. Prednisolone is used in a dose of 1 mg/kg for a period of 2–4 weeks, followed by a gradual dose reduction thereafter. Intravenous immunoglobulin gamma (IVIgG) is administered at a dose of 1 g/kg for 1–5 days, while Rh_0 (D) immunoglobulin is used exclusively in Rh-positive patients in a single dose of 50–75 μg/kg. In patients who are refractory to initial therapy, treatment options include splenectomy, rituximab (anti-CD20 monoclonal antibody), and thrombopoietin receptor agonists (romiplostim or eltrombopag) [1, 3, 4, 8]. Transfusion of platelet concentrate does not increase platelet count considering the etiopathogenesis of this disease and their rapid destruction. Platelet count can be raised preoperatively by IVIgG administered along with platelet transfusion, which in this case will have a limited effect [1].

A large number of medications can trigger immune processes that lead to thrombocytopenia (see Sect. 7.1.4).

Thrombotic thrombocytopenic purpura (TTP) and hemolytic-uremic syndrome (HUS) are classified into the category of thrombotic thrombocytopenic microangiopathies characterized by thrombocytopenia, microangiopathic hemolytic anemia with laboratory signs of hemolysis, and microvascular thrombosis [4]. TTP and HUS were previously considered the same disease, but today they are clearly differentiated, with TTP primarily associated with neurological and HUS with renal symptoms. TTP is characterized with thrombocytopenia, hemolytic anemia, fever, renal impairment, and neurological symptoms such as seizures, stroke, and altered consciousness. Bleeding is usually present as bruises on the skin, epistaxis, and hematuria. TTP is associated with inherited deficiency of metalloproteinase ADAMTS13 (Upshaw-Schulman syndrome), or the etiology of TTP is idiopathic caused by an autoimmune mechanism due to antibodies to ADAMTS13 [4]. Idiopathic form is more common in women and can occur in patients with SLE and HIV infection or in pregnancy. The metalloproteinase ADAMTS13 is an enzyme that cleaves VWF multimers. The absence of this enzyme results in the presence of large molecules of VWF that further leads to pathological platelet adhesion and aggregation, formation of thrombi, and clogging of small blood vessels (microangiopathy) in different organs. If the disease is not recognized in time, the mortality rate is extremely high, ranging from 85% to 100% [1, 4]. Plasmapheresis has significantly reduced mortality rate to 10–30%. In addition to plasma exchange, therapy includes rituximab and anti-CD20 monoclonal antibody, as well as the use of corticosteroids in idiopathic TTP [4].

HUS is a syndrome with acute renal insufficiency, microangiopathic hemolytic anemia, and thrombocytopenia that affects children and adults. In children, the disease is often preceded by hemorrhagic diarrhea, and *Escherichia coli O 157* is frequently isolated. There are also atypical forms of the disease that have a genetic basis and are usually associated with a more severe clinical presentation. Dialysis is a treatment of choice, whereas plasmapheresis does not significantly alter the course of the disease, as it does in TTP. Compared to TTP, mortality rate from HUS is lower and it is around 5% [4].

Thrombocytopenia in disseminated intravascular coagulation (DIC) is the consequence of platelet consumption in thrombotic lesions. DIC is a condition in which procoagulant factors outweigh anticoagulant ones, leading to intravascular fibrin formation and deposition, resulting in widespread vascular thrombosis and consequent damage to multiple organs. DIC is commonly seen in sepsis, usually caused by gram-negative bacteria, malignant diseases, severe head injuries, gynecological complications, immune diseases, incompatible blood transfusions, and snake bites. The underlying pathophysiological mechanism of the condition involves uncontrolled thrombin generation with suppression of physiological anticoagulant mechanisms, accompanied by pathological fibrinolysis. Multiple thromboses cause damage to numerous organs, while consumptive coagulopathy and thrombocytopathy lead to hemorrhagic syndrome and severe bleeding in the skin (purpura fulminans), mucous membranes, gastrointestinal system, urinary tract, lungs, and

CNS. The diagnosis is made based on clinical manifestations of the disease and laboratory tests that show prolonged PT and aPTT, thrombocytopenia, presence of fragmented erythrocytes (schistocytes), and elevated fibrin-degradation products, which are considered one of the most sensitive laboratory tests. Mortality rate in DIC is extremely high, due both to the underlying disease and associated complications. Treatment includes management of the underlying disease, control of hemodynamic parameters, and respiratory support. In the treatment of hemorrhagic complications, fresh frozen plasma is administered, while in the case of severe thrombocytopenia, platelet concentrate is used. In patients with multiple thromboses, treatment includes the use of anticoagulant drugs, heparin, antithrombin concentrate, and antifibrinolytics (AF) [1, 9].

Heparin-induced thrombocytopenia is described in Sect. 7.1.5.

7.1.4 Thrombocytopenia Caused by Infection and Drugs

Among the etiological factors of thrombocytopenia, infections and the use of certain pharmaceutical agents are of particular importance due to high prevalence of these thrombocytopenias and possibility to induce severe clinical manifestations. Therefore, infection-induced and drug-induced thrombocytopenias deserve to be addressed in a separate chapter.

Thrombocytopenia caused by infection is the most common non-iatrogenic form of thrombocytopenia. It occurs after viral and bacterial infections due to decreased production or shortened lifespan of platelets. In pediatric population, infections, most commonly of viral origin, can trigger immunological processes that lead to the development of thrombocytopenia. This type of disorder typically has a favorable prognosis and resolves spontaneously. In some infections, such as HIV, thrombocytopenia is a result of both increased degradation and decreased production of platelets in the bone marrow. A systemic infection may be accompanied by a hemorrhagic syndrome due to isolated thrombocytopenia but also by a more severe condition resulting from consumptive coagulopathy or DIC.

Thrombocytopenia caused by drugs may be expected during the use of chemotherapeutic agents, but it can also develop as a consequence of less predictable adverse effects of many other medications, supplements, and herbal preparations. The drugs most commonly associated with thrombocytopenia are shown in Table 7.1. The number of drugs that can induce thrombocytopenia is large, and in cases of thrombocytopenia that cannot be attributed to any apparent cause, the drug currently being administered should stop being prescribed and, if possible, replaced with an alternative. The mechanism underlying drug-induced thrombocytopenia is highly variable and involves either decreased platelet production or accelerated platelet destruction.

Drug-Induced Suppression of Platelet Production

Drugs that cause thrombocytopenia by decreasing their production in the bone marrow do not usually affect only the platelet lineage but also cause pancytopenia due to myelosuppressive effect. These drugs are busulfan, cis-platinum,

Table 7.1 Medications most commonly associated with thrombocytopenia

Medication	Group of medications	Mechanism
Antiplatelet drugs	Abciximab Eptifibatide Tirofiban	DITP
Antiarrhythmic agents	Quinidine	DITP
Antibiotics	Penicillins Cephalosporins Flucloxacillin Piperacillin Rifampin Sulfonamides Trimethoprim--sulfamethoxazole Vancomycin	DITP
Oxazolidinone antibiotics	Linezolid	Dose-dependent bone marrow suppression
Antiparasitics	Quinine	DITP
Anticonvulsants	Carbamazepine Phenytoin	DITP
Anticonvulsants	Valproic acid	Dose-dependent bone marrow suppression
Chemotherapeutics	Busulfan Cis-platinum Cyclophosphamide Cytosine arabinoside Methotrexate 6-Mercaptopurine Others	Dose-dependent bone marrow suppression
Chemotherapeutics	Oxaliplatin	DITP
Disease-modifying anti-rheumatic dugs	Gold compounds	DITP that may persist after the drug is stopped
Parenteral anticoagulants	Heparin	Drug-dependent antibodies that are also associated with thrombosis
Anti-CD20 monoclonal antibody	Rituximab	DITP
Vaccines	MMR	DITP that may persist after the drug is stopped

DITP drug-induced immune thrombocytopenia

cyclophosphamide, cytosine arabinoside, methotrexate, 6-mercaptopurine, and others. The severity of thrombocytopenia is usually the decisive criterion regarding the drug's dosage [1, 10]. The treatment of thrombocytopenia induced by chemotherapeutic and immunosuppressive agents includes the use of thrombopoietin receptor agonists, interleukin 11, and platelet transfusion when the platelet count falls below 10×10^9/L.

There are only few drugs that act selectively on megakaryocytes and, as such, can cause thrombocytopenia without pancytopenia. Pharmaceutical agents that may have such an effect include anagrelide, alcohol, estrogens, interferons, histone deacetylase inhibitors, imatinib mesylate, linezolid, and tedizolid [10].

Drug-Induced Thrombocytopenia Due to Increased Platelet Destruction
Pharmaceutical agents can cause increased platelet destruction by immunological or non-immunological mechanisms.

Non-immunologically mediated increased platelet destruction caused by drugs can arise by different mechanisms. The most common drugs that cause thrombocytopenia in this way are desmopressin (DDAVP) applied in persons with VWD; hematopoietic growth factors (granulocyte-macrophage colony-stimulating factor, granulocyte colony-stimulating factor, macrophage colony-stimulating factor); tumor necrosis factor-α and interferon-γ applied in combination for the treatment of Ewing's sarcoma; interleukin-2 applied as immunotherapy in patients with malignant diseases; protamine sulfate and heparin antagonist; amrinone and type III phosphodiesterase inhibitor, used in the therapy of heart failure; and trastuzumab and monoclonal antibody, used in the therapy of breast cancer [10].

Drug-induced immunologically mediated platelet destruction or drug-induced immune thrombocytopenia (DITP) can be caused by numerous medications. DITP is caused by accelerated platelet degradation by immunologically mediated mechanisms. The mechanisms underlying DITP are heterogeneous and often not fully elucidated. The explanation for most of these mechanisms involves the presence of natural antibodies in circulation, which under normal circumstances do not react with the platelet membrane. Following exposure to a specific drug, either the platelet surface is altered or antibodies are modified, triggering an immune response [10–12].

1. "Quinine-type" DITP is characterized by the formation of drug-dependent autoantibodies against platelets, which require the presence of the drug in plasma. In the absence of the drug, the antibodies are nonreactive, although present in the plasma. The mechanism is not sufficiently clarified considering that there is no covalent linkage between the drug and the platelet membrane. It is believed that the underlying mechanism involves the binding of the drug to the antibody, which subsequently reacts with the platelet membrane. Another proposed mechanism involves the alteration of specific molecules on the platelet membrane, most commonly the GpIIb/IIIa or GpIb receptors, which then become targets for antibody binding. Drugs that most commonly cause this type of sensitivity reaction are quinine, quinidine, ceftriaxone, piperacillin, rifampin, sulfamethoxazole, vancomycin, phenytoin, carbamazepine, nonsteroidal anti-inflammatory drugs, and many others [1, 10, 11]. This type of DITP is considered as the most common. Thrombocytopenia usually develops a few weeks after the drug initiation, or during repeated exposure. Discontinuation of the drug results in normalization of the platelet count within 7–10 days [1].
2. Hapten-induced antibody DITP occurs when the drug binds covalently to the platelet membrane, most common to GpIIb/IIIa or GpIb receptors, and acts as a hapten against which antibodies are produced. The antibodies are primarily directed against the drug-platelet complex, which clearly distinguishes this type of sensitivity reaction from the "quinine-type." This type of thrombocytopenia also depends on the presence of the drug in plasma and can occur after treatment with penicillin and some cephalosporins [1, 10, 11].

3. DITP by ligand-mimetic fibrinogen receptor antagonists can develop after the use of antiplatelet drugs, tirofiban and eptifibatide. These drugs are platelet GpIIb/IIIa antagonists but can cause acute thrombocytopenia as a side effect. Following the binding of the drug to the receptor, a modification occurs on the platelet surface, which triggers an immune process and a reaction of preexisting antibodies. This type of sensitivity reaction can occur within 24 h after initiation of the drug therapy [10, 11].
4. Drug-specific thrombocytopenia is caused by abciximab, an antagonist of GpIIb/IIIa platelet receptor that blocks the binding of fibrinogen to the activated integrin. The antibodies most likely recognize murine sequences incorporated into the chimeric (mouse-human) structure of the drug. Similar to ligand-mimetic fibrinogen receptor antagonists, abciximab causes thrombocytopenia within a few hours after drug initiation. However, thrombocytopenia can also develop later, 5–10 days after starting the treatment. Sensitivity reaction can be observed after the first, but also after repeated use of the drug [10, 11].
5. Induction of platelet-specific autoantibodies is most often associated with the use of gold preparation. The exact mechanism of the formation of these platelet autoantibodies is not fully clarified, but it is believed to be similar to the mechanism by which some antihypertensive drugs, such as methyldopa, cause autoimmune hemolytic anemia. Autoantibodies are most commonly directed toward GpIIb/IIIa receptors, although they may also target other glycoprotein receptors on the surface of platelets. Drugs that most commonly cause this type of thrombocytopenia are gold, procainamide, and levodopa. This type of sensitivity reaction continues even when the drug is discontinued [10, 11].
6. Immune complex-mediated thrombocytopenia is characterized by the formation of an immune complex through the interaction of the drug, platelet factor 4 (PF 4), and antibody, which subsequently activates platelets via Fc receptors [10, 11]. The pathogenesis of heparin-induced thrombocytopenia can be partially explained by this mechanism (see Sect. 7.1.5).

Amiodarone-associated thrombocytopenia, thrombocytopenia in patients treated with monoclonal antibodies, and protamine-associated thrombocytopenia are sometimes referred to as distinct types of DITP [10].

Numerous drugs may be potential causative agents of drug-induced thrombocytopenia, and the list of implicated drugs is subject to continuous updates. Most patients with DITP develop symptoms within 2 weeks of initiating therapy with a new drug or following reexposure to a drug that had been previously discontinued. Drugs that are taken daily over a prolonged period of time are rarely the cause of DITP. Thrombocytopenia develops abruptly and it is usually severe (platelet count $<20 \times 10^9$/L). Common clinical signs of bleeding involve bleeding gums, petechiae and purpura on the skin, and hematuria or gastrointestinal bleeding [10–12]. When the platelet count falls below 5×10^9/L, hemorrhagic bullae may develop on the buccal mucosa [10].

Laboratory findings indicate severe thrombocytopenia, which may also be accompanied by hemolytic anemia and neutropenia due to the development of antibodies against these blood components. The detection of drug-dependent antibodies that react with platelets is a reliable method for establishing the diagnosis; however, such tests are neither commonly performed in routine clinical practice, nor it is possible to detect antibodies for all drugs. False-negative results may occur due to the formation of antibodies to drug metabolites, which should also be taken into consideration during laboratory testing and diagnosis [10–12]. In the cases of thrombocytopenia that are dependent on the presence of the drug in the body, normalization of the platelet count after discontinuation of the drug is usually a sufficient criterion for the diagnosis. In patients treated with several recently introduced drugs, identifying the medication responsible for causing DITP can be challenging.

The primary therapeutic approach involves discontinuing the medication suspected of causing thrombocytopenia. Discontinuation of the drug leads to the cessation of bleeding complications within a day or two, while platelet count typically normalizes within several days. Patients should be informed that hypersensitivity to the drug is permanent and the causative drug should be avoided. Corticosteroids and IVIgG are also used in the treatment. Unlike the use in ITP, corticosteroids are less effective in DITP. In cases of significant thrombocytopenia accompanied by severe bleeding, platelet transfusion is administered; however, its effect may be limited as long as antibodies remain present in the plasma [10–12].

7.1.5 Heparin-Induced Thrombocytopenia

Thrombocytopenia caused by heparin can be nonimmune or immune-mediated. Nonimmune heparin-associated thrombocytopenia (previously referred to as type I) is caused by the direct binding of heparin to platelets, leading to their mild activation and the formation of platelet aggregates [11, 13]. Thrombocytopenia is moderate and usually occurs shortly after the initiation of therapy.

Immunologically mediated heparin-induced thrombocytopenia (HIT), previously referred to as HIT type II, is usually distinguished from other drug-induced thrombocytopenias. It is considered the most common DITP with an estimated incidence in the range of 0.1–5% [13]. The platelet count is rarely below 20×10^9/L, indicating that this type of thrombocytopenia is less associated with bleeding risk and more with an increased risk of thrombosis [1, 4, 11]. HIT is far more common in patients treated with unfractionated heparin (UFH) than in those treated with low molecular weight heparins (LMWHs). The underlying mechanism involves the formation of immune complexes between anti-PF4 antibodies and the heparin/PF4 complex. This complex activates platelets, monocytes, and endothelial cells, leading to consumptive thrombocytopenia [1, 13]. Many patients treated with heparin develop antibodies to the heparin/PF4 complex, but not all are affected by HIT. Up to 50% of individuals affected by HIT will develop thrombosis [1, 4, 11].

Venous thrombosis in the form of deep vein thrombosis and pulmonary embolism is far more common, though arterial events such as stroke, myocardial infarction, and microvascular thrombosis may also occur [13]. HIT usually occurs between 5 and 10 days after heparin administration. The timing of disease onset, along with thrombocytopenia, thrombosis, and other clinical manifestations such as skin lesions, is one of the diagnostic criteria [4, 11, 13]. HIT may occur before day 5 in patients who have been treated with heparin within the past 100 days, the period of time during which the antibodies against the heparin/PF4 complex can persist in the circulation. Rarely, HIT may develop several days following the cessation of heparin therapy [4, 11]. In this form of so-called delayed-onset HIT, antibodies can be detected in the plasma.

The diagnosis of HIT is based on clinical manifestations and laboratory testing. Laboratory testing includes detection of anti-PF4 antibodies using the enzyme-linked immunosorbent assay (ELISA) method, as well as platelet functional assays, such as serotonin release assay [4, 11, 13]. Laboratory tests should be interpreted with caution considering that many patients who develop antibodies to heparin/PF4 complex do not develop HIT.

HIT is associated with increased risk of both venous and arterial thrombosis. Deep vein thrombosis and pulmonary embolism are more common compared to arterial thrombosis. Early recognition of the disease is of great importance. The treatment of HIT involves replacing heparin with a non-heparin anticoagulant assessing the risk of bleeding versus the risk of thrombosis. Heparin is most commonly replaced with short-acting direct thrombin inhibitors (argatroban, bivalirudin, desirudin, and lepirudin), with fondaparinux or danaparoid [1, 4, 13]. Due to the high risk of thrombosis, prophylactic use of oral anticoagulant drugs should be considered. In patients with thrombosis, vitamin K antagonists (VKAs) or direct oral anticoagulant therapy is used for at least 3–6 months [4].

7.2 Thrombocytosis

Thrombocytosis and thrombocythemia are conditions characterized by increased platelet count. The most common causes are iron deficiency, reactive thrombocytosis due to inflammation or malignant disease, and myeloproliferative processes such as essential thrombocythemia or polycythemia vera [4]. Therefore, in case of an increased platelet count, diagnosis should primarily be directed toward the aforementioned conditions and diseases. An elevated platelet count is often accompanied by functional platelet defects. Thrombocytosis may pose risk for thrombosis. Markedly elevated platelet count, as seen in patients with myeloproliferative disorders, may be associated with an increased risk of bleeding due to acquired VWD and platelet binding to VWF with consequent reduction of its plasma concentration [4, 7].

7.3 Platelet Function Disorders

Platelet function disorders (thrombocytopathies) can be either congenital or acquired and result from impaired platelet adhesion, activation, granule secretion, or aggregation. Acquired platelet function disorder is usually intentionally caused by the use of antiplatelet drugs. It may also occur as an adverse reaction to high doses of penicillin, in association with certain conditions such as uremia, or as a part of myelodysplastic and myeloproliferative syndromes [4]. Inherited platelet function disorders are among the most common inherited bleeding disorders, but due to their typically mild clinical presentation, they often remain undiagnosed. The use of antiplatelet agents and dental management of these patients will be separately described (see Chaps. 25 and 26), while this chapter will discuss hereditary disorders with a higher risk of serious bleeding. This section will focus on the most common inherited platelet function disorders characterized by a significant bleeding risk.

Glanzmann thrombasthenia (GT) is an autosomal recessive disease caused by a deficiency or functional abnormality of the Gp IIb/IIIa receptor (integrin αIIbβ3 complex) on the platelet membrane. The integrin αIIbβ3 complex enables platelet-platelet interactions and serves as the binding site for fibrinogen, thus facilitating platelet aggregation. Defective platelet aggregation is the major cause of abnormal platelet function in GT [5–7, 14]. Additionally, dysfunction of integrin αIIbβ3 complex also impairs clot retraction. The incidence of GT is approximately one in million people, but in populations with higher rate of consanguineous marriages, the incidence can be significantly higher, reaching 1:200,000 [15, 16]. Both genes, *ITGA2B* and *ITGB3*, that encode GpIIb and GpIIIa are located on chromosome 17 (17q21) [15, 16]. Depending on the severity of the mutation, either a quantitative or qualitative defect of the αIIbβ3 complex arises, resulting in different severity of the disease and bleeding phenotype.

The disease typically manifests in the early childhood (usually by the age of 5), with potentially severe bleeding, although milder forms of GT are also possible.

Bleeding is usually mucocutaneous and manifests as bruises on the skin, purpura, epistaxis, gingival bleeding, bleeding from the gastrointestinal system, menorrhagia, and bleeding after trauma and surgical procedures, including tooth extraction. Less common forms of bleeding include hemarthroses and CNS bleeding [5, 7, 15]. The following tests are used for the diagnosis of GT: CBC, peripheral blood smear, light transmission aggregometry (LTA), platelet release reaction, and flow cytometry (FC). FC is used to assess the expression of glycoproteins on the platelet membrane. PFA-100 closure times and BT are usually prolonged. These tests are not commonly used due to poor sensitivity and specificity. Platelet morphology is normal, and platelet count is typically on the lower end of normal or with a mild decrease that may sometimes be observed. Ristocetin-induced platelet aggregation is normal, whereas platelet aggregation to physiological agonists (ADP, arachidonic acid, collagen, and thrombin) is absent or decreased [6, 15, 16]. FC using monoclonal antibodies CD41 and CD61 shows the absence of αIIbβ3 (<5%; type 1) or reduced expression of αIIbβ3 (5–20%; type 2) or normal expression of αIIbβ3, but with functional abnormality (>20%; type 3) [6].

Bernard-Soulier syndrome (BSS) is inherited autosomal recessive disease with an incidence of one in million. The incidence can be higher in populations where consanguineous marriages are common [16]. The disease is caused by a deficiency of GpIb-IX-V complex, which consists of four transmembrane proteins: GpIbα, GpIbβ, GpIX, and pPV. These proteins are encoded by the genes *GP1BA* (located on chromosome 17p13.2), *GP1BB* (chromosome 22q11.21), *GP9*, and *GP5* (cytogenetic location 3q21.3 and 3q29, respectively). Mutations have been identified in the genes *GP1BA*, *GP1BB*, and *GP9*, but not in the gene *GP5* [5]. These mutations can be monoallelic (mBSS) or biallelic (bBSS). mBSS form is less common and associated with milder clinical symptoms. It was previously referred to as Mediterranean thrombocytopenia, and it is inherited as autosomal dominant disorder [6, 16]. Platelet membrane receptor GpIb-IX-V is a binding site for VWF, which serves as a link between platelets and the exposed subendothelium following vascular injury.

The deficiency of GpIb-IX-V complex on the platelet membrane primarily leads to a defect in platelet adhesion but also impairs thrombin-induced platelet activation and platelet production in the bone marrow, resulting in macrothrombocytopenia and prolonged BT [5–7, 16]. The disease typically presents in the early childhood with mucocutaneous bleeding, although later onset may occur, especially in heterozygous individuals (mBSS). Bleeding manifests as frequent epistaxis, gingival bleeding, cutaneous bleeding, purpura, menorrhagia, and bleeding following trauma or surgical procedures. Hemarthroses and spontaneous intracranial bleeding are not common [5–7, 14, 16].

CBC in patients with BSS typically reveals mild to moderate thrombocytopenia, while peripheral blood smear shows the presence of macrothrombocytes. Platelet count in the same individual can fluctuate with time. PFA-100 closure times and BT are prolonged. LTA testing shows reduced response to ristocetin, which is not corrected by adding plasma. This distinguishes BSS from VWD. Platelet aggregation to ADP, arachidonic acid, collagen, and thrombin is normal [6, 16]. Due to the reduced number of platelets, LTA in some cases may yield unreliable results. FC using monoclonal antibodies CD42a (GpIX) and CD42b (GpIbα) can confirm the diagnosis of the disease [6, 16]. Considering that GT and BSS are inherited disorders, genetic analyses can confirm the presence of these diseases in multiple affected family members.

Platelet storage pool disorder is an autosomal dominant inherited disease characterized by the defect in the formation of granules in platelets or impaired secretion of granule contents (secretion platelet defects). δ-Granules or α-granules or both may be affected. Bleeding symptoms are usually mild [4].

The treatment of inherited platelet function disorders depends on the severity of the disease. Routine prophylaxis is not usually indicated. Treatment is limited to bleeding prophylaxis prior to surgical procedures, as well as treatment of uncontrolled bleeding. Mucosal bleeding in mild forms responds well to therapy with AF and local hemostasis measures [4, 6, 15, 16]. Although occasionally used, DDAVP plays a limited role in the preoperative management of patients with GT and BSS [16]. Transfusions of platelet concentrates are used in severe forms of the disease, severe bleeding complications and bleeding unresponsive to AF therapy, as well as prior to surgical procedures. Human leukocyte antigen (HLA)-matched platelet concentrate is most commonly used to prevent the risk of immunization [4, 6, 15, 16]. At the time of initial diagnosis in all patients, HLA typing and HLA antibody screening should be performed. In patients who are refractory to platelet transfusions or have antibodies to platelets (to HLA and/or to αIIβ3), activated recombinant VII coagulation factor (rVIIa) is used [15, 16]. Stem cell transplantation is successful in some cases of GT and BSS, but the risks associated with this treatment should be considered [6, 15, 16]. Gene therapy is still in its early stages and may be future direction in the treatment of patients with GT and BSS.

7.4 Clinical Manifestations and the Diagnosis of Platelet Number and Function Disorders

In the clinical presentation of patients with thrombocytopenia or a functional platelet disorder, mucocutaneous bleeding predominates. The most common symptoms are epistaxis, menorrhagia, bleeding in the oral cavity and gastrointestinal tract, skin bruises (Fig. 1.1a, b, c), and prolonged bleeding after trauma or surgical procedures. Spontaneous bleeding is unlikely when the platelet count exceeds 30×10^9/L but is commonly observed when the count falls below 10×10^9/L. It is important to note that certain types of thrombocytopenia, such as HIT, TTP, and HUS, are associated with an increased risk of thrombosis.

The diagnosis begins with obtaining a detailed medical history. Medical history should include data regarding medications, with particular attention to recently introduced drugs [10]; recent acute viral infections in children or chronic infections such as HIV or hepatitis C in adults; symptoms of the diseases and conditions that may lead to thrombocytopenia, including liver and kidney diseases, malignancies, myeloproliferative disorders, alcoholism, and malnutrition [1]; and family history when hereditary platelet disorders, such as GT and BSS, are suspected.

Thrombocytopenia with pancytopenia is suggestive of an underlying bone marrow disorder and can be seen in myelodysplastic syndromes, acute leukemias, nutritional deficiencies, or the use of chemotherapeutic agents. Isolated thrombocytopenia can be inherited, drug-induced, resulting from autoimmune diseases, such as ITP, seen in pregnancy and in patients with liver dysfunction [4].

Clinical examination may reveal signs of mucocutaneous bleeding. Cutaneous lesions typically occur on dependent areas of the body, most commonly on the lower extremities. Depending on the size, lesions are classified as petechiae (up to 3 mm in diameter), purpura (3–10 mm), and ecchymoses (>10 mm) [1]. The lesions are usually flush with the skin and do not blanch under pressure, which distinguishes them from those seen in vasculopathies. Lesions in the oral cavity are typically described as wet purpura [1, 4]. The spleen should also be palpated, and spleen size should be assessed to rule out splenomegaly.

The diagnosis is confirmed by laboratory findings. Laboratory tests include CBC, peripheral blood smear, BT, and coagulation tests PT and aPTT. In addition to a reduced platelet count, a CBC may indicate anemia and abnormalities in the white cell count, which is important for further diagnostic evaluation, including bone marrow biopsy. Bone marrow biopsy is also indicated in patients over the age of 60 with isolated thrombocytopenia to exclude myelodysplastic syndrome [1, 4]. In the case of thrombocytopenia, a peripheral blood smear is crucial in determining the etiology of the disease. Firstly, pseudothrombocytopenia must be excluded especially in cases of thrombocytopenia without clinical findings. Pseudothrombocytopenia may occur when ethylenediaminetetraacetic acid (EDTA) is used as an anticoagulant, as it can cause platelet agglutination in vitro. It can be excluded by using an alternative anticoagulant, such as sodium citrate or heparin [1, 4]. Assessment of platelet size and morphology is of great importance. For example, normal-sized platelets are seen in ITP, splenomegaly, drug-induced and infection-induced thrombocytopenia, and GT and large platelets in BSS: small platelets in Wiskott-Aldrich syndrome and X-linked thrombocytopenia [5].

BT is prolonged in patients with disorders of platelet count and function. Due to the limitations of this test, platelet function assays, such as LTA and FC, are used to assess platelet functionality [6, 16]. PT and aPTT are used to exclude the presence of coagulation disorders. Additional diagnostic tests include detection of liver diseases, HIV and hepatitis C infection, SLE, determination of heparin/PF4 antibodies, ADAMTS13 activity levels, and others [1]. Genetic testing is of great importance in patients with suspected inherited platelet disorders.

7.5 Platelet Concentrate Transfusion

The treatment of thrombocytopenia depends on the severity of the condition and the underlying cause. Platelet transfusion is used therapeutically in cases of active bleeding in patients with low platelet count or patients with disorders of platelet function. Prophylactic platelet transfusion is used to reduce the risk of spontaneous bleeding in patients with a very low platelet count ($<10 \times 10^9$/L) and to prevent hemorrhagic events in patients with thrombocytopenia and severe inherited platelet function disorders undergoing invasive procedures [9, 17]. Given the therapeutic relevance of platelet transfusion for invasive procedures, including oral surgery, the fundamental principles of this therapeutic approach will be presented in this chapter.

Platelet concentrate can be obtained either from whole blood or by apheresis. A single unit of platelet concentrate, prepared from a unit of the whole blood of a random donor, increases the platelet count by approximately 5–10 $\times$ 10^9/L. The usual dose in an adult is four to six units of the whole blood-derived platelets [1, 7]. This method of preparing platelet concentrate is cheaper and faster, but the blood units are obtained from several donors, thus exposing a patient to a higher risk of blood-borne viral infections and allergic reaction. The second method of obtaining platelet concentrate is through platelet apheresis. The concentrate is collected from a single donor, either randomly selected or HLA-compatible, thereby reducing the risk of alloimmunization and transmission of viral infections. The method involves passing the donor's blood through an automated cell separator, which separates platelets and plasma, while the red blood cells are returned to the donor's circulation. Single unit of apheresis-derived platelets is equivalent to four to six units' pool of whole blood-derived platelets and increases the platelet level by 30–50 $\times$ 10^9/L [1]. Platelet count is determined both before and immediately after platelet transfusion to evaluate the effectiveness of therapy before invasive procedure. Platelet count increases immediately after the transfusion, followed by a gradual decline over the next 3 days [1]. Preoperative platelet transfusion should be given immediately before the procedure and often after the procedure due to the rapid consumption and sequestration of platelets [7]. The total dose and duration of therapy depend on the clinical condition of the patient and indications for the treatment, prophylactic or therapeutic platelet transfusions.

A low platelet count is a relative contraindication for invasive medical procedures. Usual current practice is to correct thrombocytopenia with platelet transfusion prior to invasive procedures. The general recommendation is to administer platelet concentrate prior to most major surgical procedures if the platelet count is $<50 \times 10^9$/L [2, 17]. For eye surgery and neurosurgical procedures, recommended platelet count is $>100 \times 10^9$/L [2]. Although preoperative prophylactic platelet transfusion in cases of low platelet count is widely used in clinical practice and supported by recommendations in the literature [17], well-designed studies to confirm the benefits of this therapeutic approach are still lacking [2].

The most common adverse reactions following platelet concentrate transfusion include febrile transfusion reaction, allergic reactions, alloimmunization and refractoriness to platelet transfusion, sepsis due to product contamination, transfusion-related acute lung injury (TRALI), graft-versus-host disease (GvHD), transmission of blood-borne infections, and transfusion-associated circulatory overload [1, 2, 7]. Alloimmunization is the result of the development of antibodies to HLA and platelet antigens (HPA). The use of HLA-matched platelets reduces the risk of alloimmunization. In patients who already developed antibodies, the use of HLA-matched platelets can improve the transfusion response [1].

Platelet transfusion is contraindicated in consumptive thrombocytopenia, such as TTP and HIT, due to the risk of thrombosis. ITP is a relative contraindication, as transfused platelets are rapidly destroyed by autoimmune mechanisms. In patients with ITP, first-line therapy involves high-dose corticosteroids and IVIgG, while platelet concentrate is used for achieving hemostasis in active hemorrhagic events [1, 3, 4, 8]. If platelet transfusion is contraindicated or adverse reactions occur, alternative therapeutic options should be considered, depending on etiopathogenesis of the platelet count or function disorders [2].

References

1. Braidy HF. Review of thrombocytopenia and perioperative management in dentistry. In: Szumita RP, Szumita PM, editors. Hemostasis in dentistry. Springer eBook; 2018. p. 39–52.
2. Estcourt LJ, Malouf R, Doree C, Trivella M, Hopewell S, Birchall J. Prophylactic platelet transfusions prior to surgery for people with a low platelet count. Cochrane Database Syst Rev. 2018;9(9):CD012779.
3. Bermudez P, Beushausen M, Horan MP. Management of inherited, acquired, and iatrogenically induced coagulopathies in oral surgery. In: A textbook of advanced oral and maxillofacial surgery, vol. 3. InTech; 2016. p. 175–210.

4. Konkle BA. Disorders of platelets and vessel wall. In section: disorders of hemostasis. In: Harrison's principles of internal medicine. 20th ed. McGraw-Hill Education eBook; 2018. p. 822–30.
5. Israels S, Schwetz N, Boyar R, McNicol A. Bleeding disorders: characterization, dental considerations and management. J Can Dent Assoc. 2006;72(9):827.
6. Palma-Barqueros V, Revilla N, Sánchez A, Zamora Cánovas A, Rodriguez-Alén A, Marín-Quílez A, González-Porras JR, Vicente V, Lozano ML, Bastida JM, Rivera J. Inherited platelet disorders: an updated overview. Int J Mol Sci. 2021;22(9):4521.
7. Scully C. Haemathology. In: Scully's medical problems in dentistry. 7th ed. Elsevier: Churchill Livingstone; 2014. p. 212–75.
8. British Committee for Standards in Haematology General Haematology Task Force. Guidelines for the investigation and management of idiopathic thrombocytopenic purpura in adults, children and in pregnancy. Br J Haematol. 2003;120(04):574–96.
9. Arruda VR, High KA. Coagulation disorders. In: Harrison's principles of internal medicine. 20th ed. McGraw-Hill Education eBook; 2018. p. 830–8.
10. Aster RH. Drug-induced thrombocytopenia. In section: Disorders of platelet number and/or function. In: Michelson AD, Cattaneo M, Frelinger A, Newman PJ, editors. Platelets. 4th ed. Cambridge: Academic Press; 2019. p. 725–39.
11. Bakchoul T, Marini I. Drug-associated thrombocytopenia. Hematology Am Soc Hematol Educ Program. 2018;2018(1):576–83.
12. Arnold D, Cucker A. Drug-induced immune thrombocytopenia. https://www.uptodate.com/contents/drug-induced-immune-thrombocytopenia. Accessed 21 Oct 2022.
13. Greinacher A, Warkentin TE, Chong BH. Heparin-induced thrombocytopenia. In section: Disorders of platelet number and/or function. In: Michelson AD, Cattaneo M, Frelinger A, Newman PJ, editors. Platelets. 4th ed. Cambridge: Academic Press; 2019. p. 741–67.
14. Little JW, Miller CS, Rhodus NL. Congenital bleeding and hypercoagulable disorders. In: Little and Falace's dental management of the medically compromised patient. 9th ed. St. Louis: Elsevier; 2018. p. 457–79.
15. Poon MC, Di Minno G, d'Oiron R, Zotz R. New insights into the treatment of Glanzmann thrombasthenia. Transfus Med Rev. 2016;30(2):92–9.
16. Grainger JD, Thachil J, Will AM. How we treat the platelet glycoprotein defects; Glanzmann thrombasthenia and Bernard Soulier syndrome in children and adults. Br J Haematol. 2018;182(5):621–32.
17. Kaufman RM, Djulbegovic B, Gernsheimer T, Kleinman S, Tinmouth AT, Capocelli KE, Cipolle MD, Cohn CS, Fung MK, Grossman BJ, Mintz PD, O'Malley BA, Sesok-Pizzini DA, Shander A, Stack GE, Webert KE, Weinstein R, Welch BG, Whitman GJ, Wong EC, Tobian AA, AABB. Platelet transfusion: a clinical practice guideline from the AABB. Ann Intern Med. 2015;162(3):205–13.

Dental Management of Patients with Thrombocytopenia

8

Branislav V. Bajkin and Alison Dougall

Box 8.1 Classification of Thrombocytopenia and Dental Considerations

1. *Impaired platelet production*

Inherited (May-Hegglin anomaly, Sebastian syndrome, Fechtner syndrome, Epstein syndrome, Bernard-Soulier syndrome, Paris-Trousseau-Jacobsen's syndrome, congenital amegakaryocytic thrombocytopenia, thrombocytopenia with absent radii, Wiskott-Aldrich syndrome, X-linked thrombocytopenia, and others)

Nutritional (iron, vitamin B12 and folate deficiency, alcoholism)

Bone marrow suppression (viral infections, drug-induced, infiltration by leukemia, myeloma, lymphoma, solid tumor bone metastasis)

2. *Increased platelet sequestration* (splenomegaly)
3. *Increased platelet destruction*

Immune-related (immune thrombocytopenic purpura, drug-induced, neonatal alloimmune thrombocytopenia, posttransfusion purpura)

Nonimmune-related (thrombotic thrombocytopenic purpura, hemolytic uremic syndrome, heparin-induced thrombocytopenia, disseminated intravascular coagulopathy)

High Importance of Prevention of Oral Diseases

Oral surgery in patients with thrombocytopenia

- Consult the patient's physician
- Check platelet count before the procedure

(continued)

B. V. Bajkin (✉)
University of Novi Sad, Faculty of Medicine, Dentistry Clinic of Vojvodina, Novi Sad, Serbia
e-mail: branislav.bajkin@mf.uns.ac.rs

A. Dougall
School of Dental Science, Trinity College Dublin, Dublin Dental University Hospital, Dublin, Ireland

B. V. Bajkin (ed.), *Bleeding Disorders and Dentistry*,
https://doi.org/10.1007/978-3-032-26713-9_8

Box 8.1 (continued)

- >30 × 10^9/L minimal platelet count for inferior alveolar nerve block
- >30 × 10^9/L minimal platelet count for dental extraction [a]
- If platelet count <30 × 10^9/L, consider treatment that will raise platelet count (treatment depends on etiology of thrombocytopenia but mostly includes platelet transfusion)
- Consider antibiotic prophylaxis in a patient taking immunosuppressive agents
- Be aware of possible life-threatening bleeding in the floor of the mouth
- Schedule a patient at the beginning of the work week
- Use of local anesthesia with vasoconstrictor
- Minimally traumatic surgical technique
- Use of local hemostatic agents and measures to control oral bleeding
- Provide a patient with postoperative instructions (avoid aspirin and other NSAIDs, soft and cold diet, phone number in case of an emergency) and regular follow-up

NSAIDs nonsteroidal anti-inflammatory drugs

[a]Platelet count >50 × 10^9/L is suggested by some authors

Dentists must be familiar with the oral manifestations of a reduced platelet count, as well as the risk of postoperative bleeding after invasive dental procedures. The prevention of oral diseases in these patients is of paramount importance.

Invasive dental procedures, such as those in the domain of oral and maxillofacial surgery, periodontology, and oral implantology, require consultation with a hematologist. The risk of bleeding primarily depends on the platelet count and the extent of the procedure, but it can also be significantly influenced by other risk factors, the presence of comorbidities, and other hemostatic disorders, such as those seen in patients with liver disease. The anatomical site of the procedure within the oral cavity is also an important factor. Procedures in the floor of the oral cavity require the particular caution due to structure of the soft tissue and the potential airway obstruction resulting from bleeding. When prescribing medications, it is important to consider that certain drugs, such as acetylsalicylic acid and other nonsteroidal anti-inflammatory drugs (NSAIDs), can affect platelet function and should be avoided in these patients. Paracetamol is considered the analgesic of choice in these patients.

Recommendations regarding dental procedures are mostly based on expert opinion and guidelines established in the field of general surgery. For most routine noninvasive dental procedures, a platelet count of ≥10 × 10^9/L [1] or ≥30 × 10^9/L [2] is recommended. For block anesthesia in dentistry, including inferior alveolar nerve block (IANB), a platelet count of ≥30 × 10^9/L is recommended [1, 2]. For dentoalveolar surgery, including tooth extraction, and periodontal procedures, such as subgingival scaling and root planning, a platelet count above 50 × 10^9/L is recommended [2, 3]. There are also slightly different recommendations suggesting that a platelet count of ≥30 × 10^9/L may be sufficient for tooth extraction [1]. For more extensive oral surgical procedures, and those commonly performed in the field of maxillofacial surgery, recommended platelet count is >80 × 10^9/L [1, 2]. Platelet transfusion is used for increasing platelet number prior to the invasive procedure (see Sect. 7.5).

Tooth extraction requires close cooperation between hematologists and dentists. The procedure should be scheduled at the beginning of the day and the start of the workweek to ensure adequate time for postoperative monitoring of the patient. Following the initial assessment of the platelet count, platelet transfusion is administered if necessary. After confirming that the platelet count has reached the desired level, the procedure should be performed as soon as possible following the transfusion. The procedure should be performed with minimal trauma and with the use of local hemostatic agents and measures (see Chap. 27), along with provided detailed postoperative instructions. Depending on the risk of postoperative bleeding, the procedure can be done in either hospital or inpatient setting. Postoperative monitoring for several hours is usually sufficient, and that is the reason why outpatient or day case care oral surgery is commonplace.

There is a limited number of studies that have evaluated the risk of bleeding in patients with thrombocytopenia following dental procedures. A recently published systematic review of the literature [3] reported that, following 73 dentoalveolar procedures performed in 49 immune thrombocytopenic purpura (ITP) patients with platelet counts ranging from 2 to 412 × 10^9/L, there were two cases (2%) of clinically significant bleeding, both registered in the same patient. The first case occurred after a single tooth extraction in a patient with platelet count of 35 × 10^9/L, and bleeding was easily controlled by using local hemostatic measures. In contrast, the second case presented as life-threatening bleeding following implant placement in the posterior region of the mandible at a platelet count of 22 × 10^9/L. The submandibular hematoma, due to airway obstruction, required an emergency tracheotomy. The authors concluded that there is insufficient data on the risk of postoperative bleeding and the risk of infection in patients with ITP and that further research is needed [3].

Fillmore et al. [4] conducted a retrospective study that included 68 patients with thrombocytopenia (platelet count <100 × 10^9/L) who underwent tooth extraction. Platelet transfusion was indicated and administered in cases where the platelet count was below 50 × 10^9/L, which was done in 32 patients. The mean platelet count of the enrolled patients was 44.6 × 10^9/L. Postoperative bleeding was observed in five patients (7.4%) with a mean platelet count of 25.8 × 10^9/L, whereas no postoperative bleeding was noted in 63 patients with a mean platelet count of 46.1 × 10^9/L. All cases of postoperative bleeding were easily controlled by local hemostatic measures. The authors concluded that tooth extraction is a safe procedure in patients with thrombocytopenia if appropriate local hemostatic measures are taken. Bleeding was more frequently observed in patients with lower platelet counts; however, no clear benefits of preoperative platelet transfusion were identified [4].

Another retrospective study [5] included 89 patients with moderate to severe thrombocytopenia (platelet count <100 × 10^9/L) who required tooth extraction. In 27 patients with a platelet count <30 × 10^9/L, prophylactic preoperative platelet transfusion was given. Postoperative bleeding was recorded in four (4.4%) patients, of which in three (3.3%) cases, bleeding was successfully managed with local hemostatic measures, while one case required postoperative platelet transfusion. The authors reported an association between the extent of the oral surgical procedure (surgical tooth extraction and extraction of multiple teeth) and the risk of postoperative bleeding; however, no effect of prophylactic platelet transfusion and the platelet count itself on the risk of postoperative bleeding was observed [5].

Recent studies, although involving a limited number of patients, suggest that the recommendations advocating a platelet count >50 × 10^9/L for tooth extraction may be unwarranted and often lead to unnecessary transfusions. In line with this, there is a conclusion of a recent systematic review of the literature which states that the recommendation regarding the minimum required platelet count >50 × 10^9/L for tooth extraction is not supported by current evidence [6]. Furthermore, it is emphasized that the risk of postoperative bleeding is not solely determined by platelet count, but also by the type and site of the oral surgical procedure, as well as the patient's history of previous bleeding [7]. A few studies [5, 8], and some guidelines [1], suggest that a platelet count of ≥30 × 10^9/L could be sufficient for safe tooth extraction. Although platelet transfusion is routinely used prophylactically in patients with low platelet counts prior to surgical procedures, there is no clear evidence in the literature regarding the extent to which such treatment reduces the risk of bleeding following invasive dental procedures [9].

The available literature on dental procedures in patients with thrombocytopenia is limited, both in terms of the number of studies and the sample sizes involved. Most studies commonly include patients with thrombocytopenia of various etiologies, and many factors that may influence the risk of postoperative bleeding are usually not considered. Further investigation through randomized controlled trials is warranted to establish evidence-based protocols for dental management of these patients.

References

1. British Committee for Standards in Haematology General Haematology Task Force. Guidelines for the investigation and management of idiopathic thrombocytopenic purpura in adults, children and in pregnancy. Br J Haematol. 2003;120(4):574–96.
2. Braidy HF. Review of thrombocytopenia and perioperative management in dentistry. In: Szumita RP, Szumita PM, editors. Hemostasis in dentistry. Springer eBook; 2018. p. 39–52.
3. van Dijk WEM, van Es RJJ, Correa MEP, Schutgens REG, van Galen KPM. Dentoalveolar procedures in immune thrombocytopenia; systematic review and an institutional guideline. TH Open. 2021;5(4):e489–502.
4. Fillmore WJ, Leavitt BD, Arce K. Dental extraction in the thrombocytopenic patient is safe and complications are easily managed. J Oral Maxillofac Surg. 2013;71(10):1647–52.

5. Sandhu S, Sankar V, Villa A. Bleeding risk in thrombocytopenic patients after dental extractions: a retrospective single-center study. Oral Surg Oral Med Oral Pathol Oral Radiol. 2020;129(5):478–83.
6. Karasneh J, Christoforou J, Walker JS, et al. World Workshop on Oral Medicine VII: Platelet count and platelettransfusion for invasive dental procedures in thrombocytopenic patients: a systematic review. Oral Dis 2019;25(Suppl1):174–81.
7. Karasneh J, Christoforou J, Walker JS, et al. World Workshop on Oral Medicine VII: platelet count and platelet transfusion for invasive dental procedures in thrombocytopenic patients: a systematic review. Oral Dis. 2019;25(Suppl 1):174–81.
8. Perdigão JP, de Almeida PC, Rocha TD, Mota MR, Soares EC, Alves AP, Sousa FB. Postoperative bleeding after dental extraction in liver pretransplant patients. J Oral Maxillofac Surg. 2012;70(3):e177–84.
9. Estcourt LJ, Malouf R, Doree C, Trivella M, Hopewell S, Birchall J. Prophylactic platelet transfusions prior to surgery for people with a low platelet count. Cochrane Database Syst Rev. 2018;9(9):CD012779.

Dental Management of Patients with Platelet Function Disorders

9

Branislav V. Bajkin and Alison Dougall

Box 9.1 Dental Considerations in Patients with Inherited Platelet Function Disorders

1. *Altered adhesion* (Bernard-Soulier syndrome, platelet-type von Willebrand disease)
2. *Altered activation* (ADP receptor P2Y12 defect, TXA_2 receptor defect)
3. *Altered secretion* (gray platelet syndrome, Paris-Trousseau syndrome, Chediak-Higashi syndrome, Hermansky-Pudlak syndrome, Quebec platelet disorder)
4. *Altered aggregation* (Glanzmann thrombasthenia)
5. *Abnormalities of membrane phospholipids/procoagulant activity* (Scott syndrome)

High Importance of Prevention of Oral Diseases

Oral surgery in patients with inherited platelet function disorders

- Consult the patient's physician
- Preoperative treatment depends on the risk of the procedure, type, and the severity of the disease and may include antifibrinolytics, DDAVP, platelet transfusion, rFVIIa
- Be aware of possible life-threatening bleeding in the floor of the mouth
- Schedule a patient at the beginning of the work week
- Use of local anesthesia with vasoconstrictor

(continued)

B. V. Bajkin (✉)
University of Novi Sad, Faculty of Medicine, Dentistry Clinic of Vojvodina, Novi Sad, Serbia
e-mail: branislav.bajkin@mf.uns.ac.rs

A. Dougall
School of Dental Science, Trinity College Dublin, Dublin Dental University Hospital, Dublin, Ireland

B. V. Bajkin (ed.), *Bleeding Disorders and Dentistry*,
https://doi.org/10.1007/978-3-032-26713-9_9

Box 9.1 (continued)

- Minimally traumatic surgical technique
- Use of local hemostatic agents and measures to control oral bleeding
- Provide a patient with postoperative instructions (avoid aspirin and other NSAIDs, soft and cold diet, phone number in case of an emergency) and regular follow-up

ADP adenosine diphosphate, *DDAVP* desmopressin, *NSAIDs* nonsteroidal anti-inflammatory drugs, *rFVIIa* recombinant factor VIIa, TXA_2 thromboxane A2

Excluding the use of antiplatelet therapy, disorders of platelet function are rare, and consequently, recommendations concerning the dental management of such patients remain limited. Dental management of patients on antiplatelet therapy is presented in Chap. 26.

It is important to emphasize that dentists can have a significant role in the diagnosis of congenital platelet function disorders, such as Glanzmann thrombasthenia (GT) and Bernard-Soulier syndrome (BSS). Gingival bleeding [1], bleeding following the exfoliation of primary teeth and the eruption of permanent teeth [2], as well as a positive family history raise suspicion on inherited platelet function disorders.

Preventive dental measures and patient education regarding the importance of good oral hygiene and regular dental checkups are of great importance. Given that gum bleeding is one of the potential manifestations of these disorders, patients should be provided with instructions on how to attempt to control the bleeding through local compression. Certain medications, primarily acetylsalicylic acid and other nonsteroidal anti-inflammatory drugs (NSAIDs), but also many others such as beta-lactam antibiotics, can affect platelet function and should be avoided in these patients. Paracetamol is recommended as the analgesic of choice in patients with platelet function disorders.

In patients with GT and BSS, routine prevention of spontaneous bleeding is not recommended. Treatment is primarily focused on prevention of bleeding during surgical interventions or in treatment of spontaneous bleeding or trauma-induced hemorrhage. Preoperative treatment depends on the type of platelet function disorder, the severity of the disease, and the risk of bleeding associated with the procedure.

The use of local hemostatic agents and measures such as wound compression, soft vacuum-formed splint, and antifibrinolytics (AF) is of great importance for bleeding control following oral surgery. Tranexamic acid (TA) is used in the form of 5% mouthwash solution every 4–6 h after the procedure. AF may also be administered systemically. TA is administered orally at a dose of 25 mg/kg every 8 h or intravenously at a dose of 10 mg/kg, while ε-aminocaproic acid (EACA) can be given orally at a dose 40–60 mg/kg every 6 h, with a maximum daily dose of 30 g.

AF can be used alone or in combination with other therapeutic approaches. In milder forms of platelet function disorders and low bleeding risk procedures, desmopressin (DDAVP) may be administered at a dose of 0.3 μg/kg (maximum dose, 20 μg), either intravenously or subcutaneously, 1 h prior to the procedure [3–6]. It is confirmed that in patients with GT and BSS, a positive effect of preoperative administration of DDAVP has not been demonstrated [7].

In patients with GT and BSS, extensive oral surgical procedures with a higher risk of postoperative bleeding require systemic treatment, primarily the preoperative use of HLA-matched platelet transfusion (see Sect. 7.5). If platelet transfusion is not used prophylactically prior to surgical procedure, it should be reserved to be used in case of bleeding that cannot be controlled by local hemostatic measures. Activated recombinant factor VII (rFVIIa) is indicated in patients who are refractory to platelet transfusion therapy or have developed antiplatelet antibodies. For oral surgery, rFVIIa is administered both preoperatively and postoperatively at a dose of 90 μg/kg, with a minimum of three doses [3, 5, 7, 8]. In case when a postoperative decrease in hemoglobin level is expected, crossmatched red blood cell units should be reserved in advance [8].

Given that GT and BSS are rare hemostatic disorders, data in the literature regarding the risk of postoperative bleeding following oral surgical interventions are very limited. The results of a multicenter retrospective study [9], aimed to assess the risk of bleeding following 829 surgical procedures, including dentoalveolar interventions, in 423 patients with inherited platelet disorders (238 with function disorders and 185 with quantitative disorders), indicate a high incidence of postoperative bleeding (19.7%). A higher bleeding rate was observed in patients with function platelet disorders (24.8%) compared to those with thrombocytopenia (13.4%). A total of 233 (28.1%) dental interventions was performed, of which in 137 cases preoperative treatment involved AF, DDAVP, platelet transfusion, rFVIIa, or combinations thereof, while in the remaining 96 cases, no treatment was used. The incidence of bleeding following dental procedures was 13.3%, including 15.7% in patients with platelet function disorders and 10.1% in those with platelet count disorders [9].

The International GT Registry reported two cases (1.5%) of postoperative bleeding following 134 dental procedures [10]. For minor surgical procedures, preoperative treatment included rFVIIa, rFVIIa + AF, platelet transfusion + AF, rFVIIa combined with platelets and AF, or AF alone—largely depending on the presence of antiplatelet antibodies. Bleeding events were recorded on the second and third day after the last dose of rFVIIa and were successfully managed with repeated administration of rFVIIa [10].

In the context of invasive dental procedures in patients with BSS, recent literature reviews highlight a significant paucity of data, with most available publications limited to case reports [6]. Guidelines for the dental management of these patients, derived from published case reports, recommended consultations with a hematologist and preoperative systematic treatment involving administration of AF, DDAVP, transfusion of HLA-matched platelets, or rFVIIa. Dental procedures should be performed with minimal trauma, applying the safest local anesthetic technique accompanied by thorough postoperative instructions and avoiding prescribing medications that affect platelet function [6].

References

1. Toygar HU, Guzeldemir E. Excessive gingival bleeding in two patients with Glanzmann thrombasthenia. J Periodontol. 2007;78(6):1154–8.
2. Forde K, Mason C, Mathias M. Prolonged bleeding after exfoliation of a deciduous tooth in a patient with Glanzmann's thrombasthenia. Haemophilia. 2012;18(2):e58–9.
3. Bermudez P, Beushausen M, Horan MP. Management of inherited, acquired, and iatrogenically induced coagulopathies in oral surgery. In: A textbook of advanced oral and maxillofacial surgery, vol. 3. InTech; 2016. p. 175–210.
4. Israels S, Schwetz N, Boyar R, McNicol A. Bleeding disorders: characterization, dental considerations and management. J Can Dent Assoc. 2006;72(9):827.
5. Valera MC, Kemoun P, Cousty S, Sie P, Payrastre B. Inherited platelet disorders and oral health. J Oral Pathol Med. 2013;42(2):115–24.
6. Tieghi Neto V, Viola VP, Júnior LAVS, Santos PSDS. Invasive procedures in the oral cavity of individuals with Bernard-Soulier syndrome: an integrative review. Spec Care Dentist. 2022;42(3):281–5.
7. Grainger JD, Thachil J, Will AM. How we treat the platelet glycoprotein defects; Glanzmann thrombasthenia and Bernard Soulier syndrome in children and adults. Br J Haematol. 2018;182(5):621–32.
8. Segna E, Artoni A, Sacco R, Giannì AB. Oral surgery in patients with Glanzmann thrombasthenia: a case series. J Oral Maxillofac Surg. 2017;75(2):256–9.
9. Orsini S, Noris P, Bury L, Heller PG, Santoro C, Kadir RA, et al. European Hematology Association-Scientific Working Group (EHA-SWG) on thrombocytopenias and platelet function disorders. Bleeding risk of surgery and its prevention in patients with inherited platelet disorders. Haematologica. 2017;102(7):1192–203.
10. Poon MC, d'Oiron R, Zotz RB, Bindslev N, Di Minno MN, Di Minno G, Glanzmann Thrombasthenia Registry Investigators. The international, prospective Glanzmann thrombasthenia registry: treatment and outcomes in surgical intervention. Haematologica. 2015;100(8):1038–44.

von Willebrand Disease

10

Branislav V. Bajkin and Ivana Urosevic

von Willebrand disease (VWD) is the most prevalent congenital bleeding disorder, resulting from a quantitative deficiency or a qualitative (structural or functional) abnormality of von Willebrand factor (VWF). The prevalence of the disease is approximately 1%; however, when considering only symptomatic cases, it ranges from about one in 1000 to one in 10,000 in the general population [1–4]. Although VWD occurs equally in males and females, clinical manifestations are more commonly observed in females, primarily due to menstrual bleeding. The mutation affects the *VWF* gene located on the short arm of chromosome 12 (12p13.3). Although rare, there are also acquired forms of the disease, in which an increased plasma clearance of VWF is caused by antibodies, cell adsorption, shear stress, or increased proteolysis.

VWF is a large glycosylated protein produced by endothelial cells, megakaryocytes, and platelets. Following initial synthesis, VWF complexes containing repeating segments (multimers) with varying molecular weights are formed. Lower molecular weight VWF multimers are released into the circulation, whereas larger multimers are stored in the α-granules of platelets and the Weibel-Palade bodies of endothelial cells [2, 5, 6]. The multimeric structure of VWF creates four binding sites: two for platelet receptors GPIb/IX/V (GpIb) and GPIIb/IIIa; a binding site for subendothelial collagen, which becomes exposed following a blood vessel injury; and a binding site for coagulation factor VIII (FVIII) [5]. VWF has a dual function, participating in both primary and secondary hemostasis. In primary hemostasis, VWF mediates platelet binding to exposed subendothelial collagen via the GPIb receptor and promotes further platelet adhesion and aggregation via the GPIIb/IIIa

B. V. Bajkin (✉)
University of Novi Sad, Faculty of Medicine, Dentistry Clinic of Vojvodina, Novi Sad, Serbia
e-mail: branislav.bajkin@mf.uns.ac.rs

I. Urosevic
University of Novi Sad, Faculty of Medicine, University Clinical Center of Vojvodina, Clinic of Hematology, Novi Sad, Serbia

B. V. Bajkin (ed.), *Bleeding Disorders and Dentistry*,
https://doi.org/10.1007/978-3-032-26713-9_10

receptor. In secondary hemostasis, VWF binds and stabilizes factor FVIII, significantly prolonging its half-life in circulation [1, 5, 7].

In most cases, clinical symptoms in persons with VWD resemble those seen in patients with disorders of platelet count or function. Clinical manifestation similar to those observed in hemophilia A is related to severe forms of VWD caused by significant qualitative or quantitative deficiencies in VWF.

Classification of von Willebrand Disease

VWD is classified into three types (type 1, type 2, and type 3), with type 2 further subdivided into four subtypes: 2A, 2B, 2M, and 2N. Types 1, 2A, 2B, and 2M are inherited in an autosomal dominant manner, whereas types 2N and 3 follow an autosomal recessive pattern of inheritance. Type 1 and type 3 occur due to partial and complete deficiency of VWF, respectively, while in type 2 the structural abnormality of VWF as its qualitative defect is the pathogenic mechanism.

Type 1 is the most common form of VWD, accounting for about 70–80% of all cases [2, 7]. It involves a partial quantitative deficiency of VWF without alterations in its structure or function. Diagnosis of quantitative VWD depends on VWF levels; if VWF levels are below 30 IU/dL, these patients should be classified as having VWD type 1. The ASH/ISTH/WFH/NHF panel recommended that individuals with a significant bleeding history and plasma levels between 30 and 50 IU/dl be classified as having type 1 vWD rather than "low vWF" [3]. The condition typically appears in later childhood, with mucosal bleeding or bleeding after trauma or surgery. Frequent epistaxis, gingival bleeding, gastrointestinal bleeding, bleeding in children after tooth extraction or tonsillectomy, easy bruising, or heavy menstrual bleeding should arouse suspicion of this disorder [1]. Not all persons with low VWF concentrations exhibit bleeding symptoms. The clinical manifestation of the disease depends on the maintenance of hemostatic balance and the challenges to which the hemostatic system has been exposed. A subset of persons presents with a significant bleeding phenotype, while others exhibit only mild or no bleeding tendency (mild bleeding phenotype), a variability that cannot be attributed solely to the degree of quantitative VWF deficiency [8].

Type 1C is a specific subtype of type 1 VWD, characterized by a faster clearance of VWF from the bloodstream, leading to lower plasma levels of the factor. For patients suspected of having type 1C VWD, a desmopressin (DDAVP) test with blood samples collected at 1 and 4 h after administration is advised to evaluate for increased VWF clearance. The response to DDAVP is more pronounced; however, due to the shorter half-life of VWF, this therapy may be less effective compared to type 1 VWD [4].

A functional defect in VWF characterizes type 2 VWD and accounts for about 15–30% of all cases of the disease. Type 2 VWD is further classified into four subtypes—2A, 2B, 2M, and 2N—which differ primarily in the type of qualitative VWF defect. In types 2A, 2B, and 2M, the binding activity of VWF to platelets and/or collagen is reduced. Type 2A VWD is characterized by a deficiency of high- and intermediate-molecular-weight VWF multimers, leading to impaired platelet adhesion and reduced binding affinity to collagen. This subtype of VWD is the most common among type 2 variants, accounting for approximately 15–20% of all VWD cases [7]. Type 2B VWD is caused by a mutation that affects the binding site of VWF to the GPIb receptor on the platelet membrane. Due to the increased affinity of VWF for platelets and accelerated platelet clearance by the reticuloendothelial system, this type is typically associated with varying degrees of thrombocytopenia. Type 2M VWD is characterized by a standard VWF structure, which distinguishes it from type 2A. This type, like type 2B, results from a mutation that affects the platelet-binding site; however, it leads to decreased VWF affinity for platelets and impaired platelet adhesion. In type 2N, the multimeric structure of VWF is not altered. There is a defect in the binding of VWF to FVIII. The half-life of FVIII is shortened, resulting in reduced plasma concentration, making this type of disorder clinically similar to hemophilia A [1, 9].

Type 3 VWD is a rare and severe form of the disorder, affecting about one to three per million people and making up roughly 5% of all cases. It is marked by an almost complete deficiency of VWF in plasma and platelets. This near-total loss of VWF in type 3 disorder is inherited in an autosomal recessive pattern, with individuals being homozygous or compound heterozygous for two nonsense mutations (null alleles). The FVIII level is reduced, dropping below 10% [1]. The disorder causes mucocutaneous bleeding, bleeding after trauma and surgery, and joint bleeding similar to that seen in individuals with hemophilia A. FVIII/VWF concentrate is used to control bleeding in these patients, with a potential risk of developing antibodies after treatment.

Acquired VWD is a rare disorder that typically occurs in patients with lymphoproliferative diseases, such as monoclonal gammopathy of undetermined significance, multiple myeloma, and Waldenström macroglobulinemia, as well as in patients with autoimmune diseases and those with aortic valve stenosis [1, 5, 10]. The disorder manifests later in life in individuals who previously had no bleeding complications and have no positive family history.

In the general population, normal plasma vWF levels range from 50 to 200 IU/dL. Lower plasma vWF levels are observed in individuals with blood group "0," approximately 25% lower than those with other blood groups [11].

Diagnosis of von Willebrand Disease

The diagnosis of VWD is established based on medical history, including positive family history, a clinical presentation characterized by recurrent bleeding episodes, and laboratory findings. They indicate decreased levels or functional activity of VWF and/or FVIII. It should be noted that different types of VWD exhibit distinct clinical manifestations; thus, a spectrum from mild to severe forms of the disease is possible. A positive family history may not be clearly evident. Bleeding typically manifests as mucocutaneous hemorrhage, while hemarthroses and more severe deep tissue bleeding are observed only in individuals with type 3 VWD.

Laboratory diagnosis of VWD includes quantitative assessment of VWF (VWF antigen, VWF:Ag), functional evaluation of VWF (VWF ristocetin cofactor activity, VWF:RCo; ristocetin-induced platelet aggregation, RIPA; VWF binding to collagen, VWF:CB; and VWF:FVIII-binding assay), assessment of coagulation activity through measurement of FVIII concentration (FVIII:C), analysis of VWF multimers, and determination of VWF propeptide levels (VWFpp) [1–4, 7]. The values of some of these tests, along with activated partial thromboplastin time (aPTT) results for specific VWD types, are shown in Table 10.1. There are also newer assays for functional evaluation of VWF, such as VWF binding to the GPIb receptor (VWF:GPIbM, VWF:GPIbR), which offer certain advantages over the traditional VWF:RCo assay [3]. Normal levels of VWF:Ag range from 0.50 to 2.0 IU/mL, while undetectable levels or levels <0.05 IU/mL are indicative of type 3 VWD. VWF levels <0.30 IU/mL, regardless of bleeding symptoms, or levels <0.50 IU/mL with

Table 10.1 Laboratory characteristics of VWD types and DDAVP response

VWD type	Cause of VWD	aPTT	VWF antigen	VWF activity	FVIII activity (FVIII:C)	VWF activity/Ag	DDAVP response
1	Partial quantitative deficiency of VWF; normal multimers	Normal or ↑	↓ to ↓↓	↓ to ↓↓	Normal to ↓	>0.7	Usually positive (↑ VWF and FVIII)
1C	Increased clearance of VWF; normal multimers	Normal or ↑	↓ to ↓↓	↓ to ↓↓	Normal to ↓	>0.7	DDAVP trial with 1- and 4-h postadministration blood work to confirm increased clearance in persons with suspected type 1C VWD[a]
2A	VWF reduced binding to platelets; deficiency of the VWF multimers	Normal or ↑	Normal to ↓	↓↓	Normal to ↓	<0.7	Variable (↑ FVIII)
2B	VWF increased affinity for platelet GPIb; loss of the VWF multimers	Normal or ↑	↓	↓↓	Normal to ↓	<0.7	Contraindicated due to thrombocytopenia
2M	Decreased VWF-dependent platelet adhesion; normal VWF multimers	Normal or ↑	↓	↓↓	Normal to ↓	<0.7	Variable, usually no response

(continued)

Table 10.1 (continued)

VWD type	Cause of VWD	aPTT	VWF antigen	VWF activity	FVIII activity (FVIII:C)	VWF activity/Ag	DDAVP response
2N	Reduced affinity for FVIII; normal VWF multimers	↑↑	↓	↓↓	Normal to ↓	<0.7	Variable, usually no response
3	VWF complete deficiency	↑↑	↓↓↓	↓↓↓	↓↓↓	N/A	No response

↓, slightly reduced; ↓↓, moderately reduced; ↓↓↓, significantly reduced

VWD von Willebrand disease, *VWF* von Willebrand factor, *aPTT* activated partial thromboplastin time, VWF:Ag activity, quantitative assessment of VWF; VWF: activity, functional assessment of VWF, assessment of the ability of VWF to bind platelets and/or collagen; *FVIII:C* the measurement of FVIII coagulant activity, *DDAVP* desmopressin, *N/A* not applicable

[a]DDAVP response requires an increase of at least >2 times the baseline VWF activity level and a sustained increase of both VWF and factor FVIII (FVIII:C) levels >0.50 IU/mL for at least 4 h

clinically manifested bleeding confirm the diagnosis of type 1 VWD [3]. In addition to laboratory evaluation, genetic testing is also performed for the diagnosis of VWD (Fig. 10.1).

Treatment of von Willebrand Disease

The treatment of VWD involves increasing the level of VWF by the use of DDAVP or FVIII/VWF concentrates, either plasma-derived or recombinant, as well as the use of antifibrinolytics (tranexamic acid, TA, or ε-aminocaproic acid, EACA) and local hemostatic agents and measures. The treatment depends on the type of VWD and severity of bleeding event or the bleeding risk of associated with an invasive procedure.

DDAVP is a synthetic derivative of the antidiuretic hormone that promotes the release of VWF and FVIII from the endothelium. It is assumed that DDAVP binds to the V2 receptor on endothelial cells, which triggers a cascade of intracellular signaling pathways involving cAMP, and leads to the release of stored VWF from Weibel-Palade bodies of the endothelial cells. The increase of FVIII concentration is presumed to result not only from its release but also from enhanced stabilization in the plasma, facilitated by its binding to VWF. DDAVP is capable of correcting only mild VWF deficiencies; thus, it is most effective in persons with type 1 VWD and generally contraindicated in type 1C VWD patients in the setting of surgery. In individuals who respond well to therapy, DDAVP induces a three- to fivefold increase in VWF and FVIII levels in plasma. DDAVP is administered parenterally, either subcutaneously or intravenously, at a dose of 0.3 μg/kg (maximum dose 15 μg) or as a high-dose intranasal spray, 150 μg for children weighing up to 50 kg, or 300 μg (150 μg in each nostril) for persons over 50 kg [1, 2, 6]. DDAVP is also used for surgical procedures with low to moderate bleeding risk, including oral surgical interventions, in persons who respond well to the therapy. The maximal

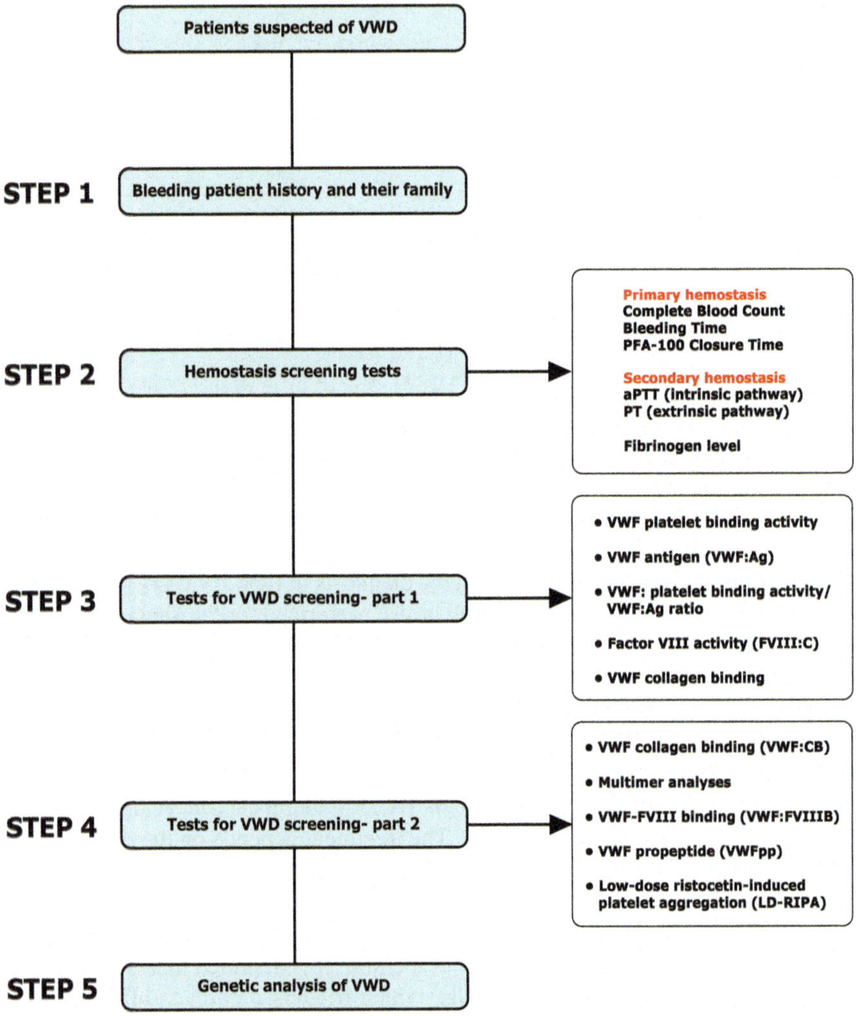

Fig. 10.1 Algorithm for the diagnosis of VWD

effect of the drug occurs approximately 30 min after intravenous administration, with a duration of action lasting 6–12 h. DDAVP is administered intranasally in cases of mild bleeding or preoperatively for minor surgery, with a maximal effect occurring approximately 2 h after administration. Depending on the individual response, the bleeding risk, and the extent of the surgical procedure, the dose of the drug may be repeated postoperatively at intervals of 12–24 h [1, 2, 7]. DDAVP can sometimes be successfully used during minor surgical procedures in some persons with type 2A, 2M, and 2N VWD (Table 10.1). The drug's effect is highly individual, making it essential before the use to verify whether the person responds to this therapy [7, 10]. The use of DDAVP in persons with type 3 VWD is ineffective, while in persons with type 2B, VWD is contraindicated, as it may worsen thrombocytopenia. The main adverse effect of DDAVP administration is hyponatremia, which typically occurs in very young or elderly individuals [1]. Other adverse effects are related to vasodilation and include tachycardia, hypotension, facial flushing, and headache.

Concentrates containing VWF are used prior to surgical procedures or in need of bleeding control in persons with type 3 and type 1C, as well as in most of those with type 2 VWD who do not respond adequately to DDAVP therapy. A WFH concentrate is also recommended for persons undergoing high-risk procedures (e.g., neurosurgical procedures), regardless of their responsiveness to DDAVP therapy [10]. There are plasma-derived FVIII/VWF concentrates in which the two factors are present in varying ratios, as well as highly purified plasma-derived VWF concentrates and recombinant VWF concentrates [2, 10]. If a highly purified VWF concentrate is used in the case of major surgical procedures or severe bleeding events, a FVIII concentrate is commonly coadministered to ensure adequate hemostatic response [10]. Plasma-derived products undergo viral inactivation processes, minimizing the risk of transmission of blood-borne infections. Plasma-derived VWF concentrates differ in their VWF:RCo activity, which may influence their clinical efficacy and dosing strategies. VWF concentrate may also be used for long-term prophylaxis, but only in persons with severe forms of VWD and frequent and severe bleeding episodes [10].

The administration of antifibrinolytic agents is of great importance in persons with VWD presenting with mucosal bleeding or those undergoing surgical procedures such as tonsillectomy or oral surgery [1]. Antifibrinolytic agents inhibit the conversion of plasminogen to plasmin. TA is most commonly used at a dose of 1 g administered orally, three times daily, for 7 days. Antifibrinolytics can also be applied locally, either as a mouth rinse solution or by direct application to the wound, alone or in combination with a local hemostatic agent (see Chap. 27).

References

1. Konkle BA. Disorders of platelets and vessel wall. In section: Disorders of hemostasis. In: Harrison's principles of internal medicine. 20th ed. McGraw-Hill Education eBook; 2018. p. 822–30.
2. Leebeek FW, Eikenboom JC. VonWillebrand's disease. N Engl J Med. 2016;375:2067–80.
3. James PD, Connell NT, Ameer B, Di Paola J, Eikenboom J, Giraud N, Haberichter S, et al. ASH ISTH NHF WFH 2021 guidelines on the diagnosis of von Willebrand disease. Blood Adv. 2021;5(1):280–300.
4. Ng C, Motto DG, Di Paola J. Diagnostic approach to von Willebrand disease. Blood. 2015;125(13):2029–37.
5. Szumita RP. Review of von Willebrand disease and perioperative management in dentistry. In: Szumita RP, Szumita PM, editors. Hemostasis in dentistry. Springer; 2018. p. 27–32.
6. Bermudez P, Beushausen M, Horan MP. Management of inherited, acquired, and iatrogenically induced coagulopathies in oral surgery. In: A textbook of advanced oral and maxillofacial surgery, vol. 3. InTech; 2016. p. 175–210.

7. Little JW, Miller CS, Rhodus NL. Congenital bleeding and hypercoagulable disorders. In: Little and Falace's dental management of the medically compromised patient. 9th ed. St. Louis: Elsevier; 2018. p. 457–79.
8. Doherty D, Lavin M, O'Sullivan JM, Ryan K, O'Connell NM, Dougall A, Byrne M, Rafferty M, Doyle MM, Di Paola J, James PD, O'Donnell JS. Management of elective procedures in low von Willebrand factor patients in the LoVIC study. J Thromb Haemost. 2021;19(3):701–10.
9. Scully C. Haemathology. In: Scully's medical problems in dentistry. 7th ed. Elsevier: Churchill Livingstone; 2014. p. 212–75.
10. Connell NT, Flood VH, Brignardello-Petersen R, Abdul-Kadir R, Arapshian A, Couper S, et al. ASH ISTH NHF WFH 2021 guidelines on the management of von Willebrand disease. Blood Adv. 2021;5(1):301–25.
11. Liang Q, Li R. Recent advances in the diagnosis of von Willebrand disease. LabMed Discov. 2024;1(2):100020.

Dental Management of Persons with von Willebrand Disease

11

Branislav V. Bajkin and Alison Dougall

Box 11.1 Dental Considerations in Patients with VWD

1. Type 1 VWD (partial quantitative VWF defect)
2. Type 2 VWD (qualitative VWF defect; four subtypes: 2A, 2B, 2M, and 2N)
3. Type 3 VWD (complete lack of VWF)

High Importance of Prevention of Oral Diseases

- Gingival bleeding is more related to poor oral hygiene and local inflammation than to the disease itself

Oral Surgery in Patients with VWD

- Consult the patient's physician
- Individualized dental treatment plan in discussion with a hematologist
- Inpatient or outpatient treatment depending on the bleeding risk of the procedure
- Perioperative hematological treatment depends on the risk of the procedure, type, and the severity of the disease and may include DDAVP, concentrate VW, and antifibrinolytics
  - DDAVP is effective in type 1 and in some patients with types 2A, 2M, and 2N VWDs
  - DDAVP responsiveness should be obtained before using DDAVP for therapeutic interventions

(continued)

B. V. Bajkin (✉)
University of Novi Sad, Faculty of Medicine, Dentistry Clinic of Vojvodina, Novi Sad, Serbia
e-mail: branislav.bajkin@mf.uns.ac.rs

A. Dougall
School of Dental Science, Trinity College Dublin, Dublin Dental University Hospital, Dublin, Ireland

B. V. Bajkin (ed.), *Bleeding Disorders and Dentistry*,
https://doi.org/10.1007/978-3-032-26713-9_11

Box 11.1 (continued)

- Concentrate VWF should be used in type 3 and type 2B VWD and in other type 2 VWD patients with lack of DDAVP efficacy
- Use of antifibrinolytics systemically and/or locally along with DDAVP or concentrate VWF
- Increase preoperatively VWF activity levels to >0.50 IU/mL with DDAVP or factor concentrate with the addition of antifibrinolytics
- For intervention in a patient with type 1 VWD with baseline VWF activity levels of >0.30 IU/mL and a mild bleeding phenotype, give TA alone over increasing VWF activity levels to >0.50 IU/mL

- Be aware of possible life-threatening bleeding in the floor of the mouth
- Schedule a patient at the beginning of the work week
- Use of local anesthesia with vasoconstrictor
- Avoid IANB; if IANB is necessary, concentrate VWF is required in type 3 VWD and DDAVP or concentrate VWF in type 2 VWD, as well as in type 1 VWD with severe bleeding phenotype
- Minimally traumatic surgical technique
- Use of local hemostatic agents and measures to control oral bleeding
- Local use of antifibrinolytics in the form of mouthwash solution may be of great importance
- For pain relief, use acetaminophen or selective C0X-2 inhibitors; avoid aspirin and other NSAIDs
- Provide a patient with postoperative instructions (soft and cold diet, phone number in case of an emergency) and regular follow-up

VWD von Willebrand disease, *VWF* von Willebrand factor, *DDAVP* desmopressin, *IANB* inferior alveolar nerve block, *COX-2* cyclooxigenase-2, *NSAIDs* nonsteroidal anti-inflammatory drugs

As in case of other bleeding disorders, the role of the dentist in VWD is to educate affected children and their parents regarding the importance of maintaining optimal oral hygiene and implementing preventive measures to minimize the risk of oral diseases. Preventive examinations and early dental interventions in childhood can reduce the need for invasive procedures, which pose a risk for persons with VWD and incurs significant costs [1].

Gingival bleeding has traditionally been cited as one of the manifestations VWD and was attributed to the disease itself. However, gingival bleeding is more often a consequence of poor oral hygiene and plaque-induced gingivitis. Recent studies have not found a correlation between VWD and gum bleeding in persons with type 1 VWD [2, 3]. In addition, neither bleeding on probing (BOP) nor gingival bleeding index (GBI) has higher values in persons with type 2 or type 3 VWD compared to a control group of subjects without a hemostatic disorder [4]. The conclusion of these studies [2–5] is that in persons with VWD, gingival bleeding is more likely a result of accumulated dental plaque, local inflammation, and periodontal disease, rather than a symptom of the underlying hematologic disorder. The conclusion of a recently published review article, based on the analysis of a very limited number of studies, is that persons with VWD do not have a greater predisposition to the development of periodontal diseases compared to healthy individuals [6].

Dental diseases such as caries and periodontal diseases are highly preventable. Adherence to proper oral hygiene practices and dietary advice are of great importance. Dentists must also be aware that the assessment of periodontal indices and professional dental cleaning in persons with VWD can be performed without significant risk of postoperative bleeding. Unlike supragingival cleaning, subgingival debridement and periodontal surgical procedures, particularly in persons with type 2 and type 3 VWD, may be associated with prolonged bleeding and may require appropriate systemic preoperative measures, as well as the use of local hemostatic agents, to minimize the risk of hemorrhage. The use of antifibrinolytics is of exceptional importance in the prevention and management of all mucosal bleeding. To minimize the risk associated with periodontal procedures, careful planning is required, including preoperative reduction of gingival inflammation through the use of antibiotics and antibacterial mouthwash solutions, as well as performing the intervention in multiple visits if necessary.

VWD is the most common inherited bleeding disorder. However, due to its mild clinical presentation particularly in type 1, it often remains undiagnosed. The extraction of a deciduous or permanent tooth often represents the first significant challenge to the hemostatic system, and post-extraction bleeding is frequently cited as one of the most common indications to consider the possibility of VWD [7, 8].

Tooth extraction or any other invasive oral surgical procedure requires close collaboration between the dentist and the hematologist.

According to the joint recommendation of the American Society of Hematology, International Society on Thrombosis and Haemostasis, National Hemophilia Foundation, and World Federation of Hemophilia, for more extensive procedures such as those in the field of maxillofacial surgery, FVIII activity and VWF activity should be maintained at levels >0.50 IU/mL for at least 3 days postoperatively [9]. For dentoalveolar surgery, including tooth extraction, the recommendation is to achieve minimum VFW activity levels >0.50 IU/mL preoperatively by using DDAVP or FVIII/VWF or VWF concentrates, with additional use of antifibrinolytics [9, 10]. In persons with type 1 VWD with baseline VWF levels >0.30 IU/mL and mild bleeding phenotype, priority should be given to the use of tranexamic acid (TA) over raising VWF activity levels to >0.50 IU/mL by the use of DDAVP or VWF-containing concentrates [9]. An individualized therapeutic approach is required for all dental procedures [9]. The use of local hemostasis agents can significantly reduce the need for systemic hemostasis measures and lower the risk of postoperative bleeding.

A limited number of studies aimed at assessing the risk of postoperative bleeding following oral surgical procedures in persons with VWD can be found in the literature. These studies usually involved a small number of participants with different types of VWD and varying bleeding phenotypes, which affects the overall risk of postoperative bleeding. Also, it can be noted that there is no consensus in the literature regarding the need for systemic hemostatic measures or the duration of DDAVP or VWF concentrate administration for tooth extraction.

A retrospective study published by Federici et al. [11] included 63 persons with different types of VWD who underwent either tooth extraction or periodontal procedures. The participants were divided into two groups based on the treatment approach: one group (30 participants) received only local hemostatic measures, TA and/or fibrin glue, while the other group (33 participants) received systemic therapy, either DDAVP or VWF/FVIII concentrate in a single preoperative dose, in addition to local measures. The therapeutic approach was determined upon agreement between the dentist and the hematologist and depended on the extent of the planned dental procedure, the type of VWD, and the presence of comorbidities. Postoperative bleeding was registered in one patient from each group (two out of 63, 3.1%) and was easily controlled using local hemostatic measures. The authors concluded that the use of local hemostatic measures can significantly reduce the need for systemic therapy and that the use of TA, fibrin glue, and DDAVP proved to be sufficient and effective in preventing postoperative bleeding after oral surgical interventions in the majority of cases (84%) [11].

There are also studies that advocate the administration of VWF concentrate both pre- and postoperatively for several days as a prevention of bleeding following oral surgical procedures. De Padua et al. [12] reported no cases of postoperative bleeding following 45 oral surgical procedures in 20 persons with different types of VWD who were treated with VWF/FVIII concentrate pre- and postoperatively according to the protocol customized for each person. Morimoto et al. [13] reported successful bleeding control in 37 cases following dental procedures in 19 persons with VWD with multiple doses of DDAVP or VWF/FVIII concentrate, depending on the type of VWD. The authors emphasized the importance of using TA in combination with DDAVP or VWF/FVIII concentrate and the need for different protocols for the extraction of primary and permanent teeth, surgical tooth extraction, and gingival bleeding [13].

In the study published by Doherty et al. [14], invasive procedures were analyzed in 60 individuals with mildly reduced VWF levels (0.30–0.50 IU/mL). A retrospective analysis conducted prior to the diagnosis of low VWF levels showed that post-extraction bleeding was reported in 62.5% (30 of 48 of persons) and that additional interventions, such as packing, wound suturing, and transfusion were required in 43.8% (23 of 48) of cases. After the diagnosis of low VWF levels, 40 dental procedures were performed, of which 34 were single tooth extractions, three multiple tooth extractions, and three root canal treatments. Preoperative prophylaxis included the use of TA at a dose of 1 g three times daily, orally or intravenously (10/40), DDAVP at a dose of 0.3 μg/kg (16/40), DDAVP + TA (13/40), and VWF concentrate + TA (1/40). Postoperative bleeding was observed in 10% (four of 40) of cases after single tooth extraction, in three cases who received prophylaxis with TA, and in one with DDAVP prophylaxis. Bleeding was successfully controlled with DDAVP in two cases, and with TA and local hemostatic measures in one case each. The authors concluded that there was insufficient evidence to support that prophylaxis with TA alone is sufficiently effective in bleeding prevention for tooth extraction in this group of persons with VWD [14].

Inferior alveolar nerve block (IANB) requires caution. Prophylaxis with FVIII/VWF concentrate is recommended, especially in the most severe forms of VWD, such as type 3 [15]. Some recommendations suggest that minor dental procedures in persons with type 1 VWD or "low VWF" that require IANB can be done with prophylaxis with DDAVP with or without TA [16].

Given that the recommendations regarding dental management of persons with type 3 VWD and hemophilia A and B mostly coincide, more detailed recommendations will be presented in Chap. 13.

References

1. Carcao MD, Seary ME, Casas M, Winter L, Stain AM, Judd P. Dental disease in type 3 Von Willebrand disease: a neglected problem. Haemophilia. 2010;16(6):943–8.
2. Weickert L, Miesbach W, Alesci SR, Eickholz P, Nickles K. Is gingival bleeding a symptom of patients with type 1 von Willebrand disease? A case-control study. J Clin Periodontol. 2014;41(8):766–71.
3. Weickert L, Krekeler S, Nickles K, Eickholz P, Seifried E, Miesbach W. Gingival bleeding and mild type 1 von Willebrand disease. Blood Coagul Fibrinolysis. 2017;28(1):19–23.
4. Epping L, Miesbach W, Nickles K, Eickholz P. Is gingival bleeding a symptom of type 2 and 3 von Willebrand disease? PLoS One. 2018;13(1):e0191291.
5. Vanduine S, Ridley K, Bashutski J, Snyder M, Powell C, Taichman S. Gingival bleeding and oral hygiene in women with von Willebrand disease (VWD): a pilot study. J Haem Pract. 2017;4:49–57.
6. Mester A, Mancini L, Marchetti E, Baciut M, Bran S, Lucaciu O, et al. The presence of periodontitis in patients with von Willebrand disease: a systematic review. Appl Sci. 2021;11(14):6408.
7. Cohen AJ, Kessler CM, Ewenstein BM, Hemophilia Research Society of North America. Management of von Willebrand disease: a survey on current clinical practice from the haemophilia centres of North America. Haemophilia. 2001;7(3):235–41.
8. Baghaie H, Forrest B, Shukla K, Liu T. Dental extraction in a patient with undiagnosed von Willebrand's disease: a case report. Aust Dent J. 2021;66(1):105–11.
9. Connell NT, Flood VH, Brignardello-Petersen R, Abdul-Kadir R, Arapshian A, Couper S, et al. ASH ISTH NHF WFH 2021 guidelines on the management of von Willebrand disease. Blood Adv. 2021;5(1):301–25.
10. Leebeek FW, Eikenboom JC. Von Willebrand's disease. N Engl J Med. 2016;375:2067–80.
11. Federici AB, Sacco R, Stabile F, Carpenedo M, Zingaro E, Mannucci PM. Optimising local therapy during oral surgery in patients with von Willebrand disease: effective results from a retrospective analysis of 63 cases. Haemophilia. 2000;6(2):71–7.
12. De Padua V, Romeo U, Santoro C, Bosco R, Baldacci E, Ferretti A, Malaspina F, Mazzucconi MG, Gaglioti D. Dental invasive procedures in von Willebrand disease outpatients treated with high purity FVIII/VWF complex concentrate (Fanhdi®): experience of a single center. Heliyon. 2020;6(2):e03426.
13. Morimoto Y, Yoshioka A, Sugimoto M, Imai Y, Kirita T. Haemostatic management of intraoral bleeding in patients with von Willebrand disease. Oral Dis. 2005;11(4):243–8.

14. Doherty D, Lavin M, O'Sullivan JM, Ryan K, O'Connell NM, Dougall A, Byrne M, Rafferty M, Doyle MM, Di Paola J, James PD, O'Donnell JS. Management of elective procedures in low von Willebrand factor patients in the LoVIC study. J Thromb Haemost. 2021;19(3):701–10.
15. Piot B, Sigaud-Fiks M, Huet P, Fressinaud E, Trossaërt M, Mercier J. Management of dental extractions in patients with bleeding disorders. Oral Surg Oral Med Oral Pathol Oral Radiol Endod. 2002;93(3):247–50.
16. Laffan MA, Lester W, O'Donnell JS, Will A, Tait RC, Goodeve A, Millar CM, Keeling DM. The diagnosis and management of von Willebrand disease: a United Kingdom Haemophilia Centre Doctors Organization guideline approved by the British Committee for Standards in Haematology. Br J Haematol. 2014;167(4):453–65.

12 Coagulopathies

Branislav V. Bajkin and Ivana Urosevic

When coagulopathies are mentioned, the first thing that usually comes to mind is an inherited deficiency of one of the coagulation factors, primarily hemophilia A (FVIII deficiency) and hemophilia B (FIX deficiency). According to data from the World Federation of Hemophilia (WFH) from 2020, it is estimated that the number of males with hemophilia is around 1,125,000, of which approximately 418,000 are estimated to have severe hemophilia [1]. Hemophilia A is far more common than hemophilia B, accounting for about 80%–85% of all hemophilia cases. In both conditions, there is a deficiency in the intrinsic coagulation pathway, resulting in a limited capacity for factor X activation and the further cascade leading to the generation of thrombin and fibrin.

Coagulopathies also include other rare bleeding disorders caused by deficiencies of coagulation factors such as FII, FV, FVII, FX, FXI, FXIII, and fibrinogen, which are predominantly inherited in an autosomal recessive manner [2]. Laboratory tests in these conditions show prolonged prothrombin time (PT) and/or activated partial thromboplastin time (aPTT), depending on the deficiency of a specific factor in the extrinsic, intrinsic, or common coagulation pathway (see Sects. 2.3 and 3.2).

Acquired coagulation disorders are more common than congenital ones and commonly arise secondary to hepatic pathology, disseminated intravascular coagulation (DIC), and vitamin K deficiency. These conditions typically involve deficiencies of several coagulation factors, and in certain cases, such as liver disease and DIC, there is concomitant disruption of primary hemostasis [2].

It is also important to highlight the possibility of developing autoantibodies to certain coagulation factors. Such antibodies, referred to as inhibitors, most

B. V. Bajkin (✉)
University of Novi Sad, Faculty of Medicine, Dentistry Clinic of Vojvodina, Novi Sad, Serbia
e-mail: branislav.bajkin@mf.uns.ac.rs

I. Urosevic
University of Novi Sad, Faculty of Medicine, University Clinical Center of Vojvodina, Clinic of Hematology, Novi Sad, Serbia

B. V. Bajkin (ed.), *Bleeding Disorders and Dentistry*,
https://doi.org/10.1007/978-3-032-26713-9_12

commonly develop through a mechanism that remains incompletely elucidated in persons with severe forms of hemophilia A and B who have previously been treated with the appropriate factor concentrate. Inhibitor development is also possible in patients with no prior history of a hemostatic disorder, occurring as a consequence of autoimmune or neoplastic diseases or arising idiopathically. The use of bovine thrombin as a local hemostatic agent can cause the formation of antibodies against thrombin [2]. In the diagnosis and treatment of these conditions, the detection and determination of inhibitor titer are of utmost importance.

12.1 Hemophilia A

Hemophilia A is a congenital coagulopathy caused by a deficiency of FVIII. It is inherited in an X-linked recessive pattern and results from a mutation in the *F8* gene, located on the long arm of the X chromosome (Xq28). The estimated prevalence of hemophilia A is 24.6 cases per 100,000 male newborns, of which 9.5 cases are severe [1]. The disease predominantly affects males, while females who carry a single mutated gene on one of the X chromosomes are carriers and may be asymptomatic or show mild symptoms. The disorder can also arise as a consequence of a de novo mutation, in which case there is no positive family history. It is estimated that de novo mutations account for approximately one-third of all cases of hemophilia [3–5].

The severity of the disorder' s clinical manifestations correlates with the circulating plasma FVIII activity without treatment. FVIII activity in plasma is expressed either as a percentage (relative to normal human plasma) or in IU (relative to an international standard for FVIII in plasma), and the FVIII reference range is 50%–150% or 50–150 IU/dL (0.5–1.5 IU/mL). Hemophilia A is classified as severe (FVIII level < 1%), moderate (FVIII level 1%–5%), and mild (FVIII level 5%–40%) (Table 12.1). The severe form of the disease is characterized by spontaneous bleeding into joints (hemarthroses), into soft tissues primarily muscles (Fig. 12.1), and into internal organs, as well as prolonged bleeding following minor surgical

Table 12.1 Clinical manifestations of hemophilia A and B in relation to the concentrations of FVIII and FIX

Severity of the disease	FVIII/FIX levels	Clinical feature
Severe	<1 IU/dl or <1% of normal	Frequent spontaneous bleeding into the joints and muscles; massive bleeding after minor trauma and surgical procedures
Moderate	1–5 IU/dl or 1%–5% of normal	Occasional spontaneous bleeding into the joints and muscles; prolonged bleeding after minor trauma and surgical procedures
Mild	5–40 IU/dl or 5%–40% of normal	Rare spontaneous bleeding, prolonged bleeding after serious trauma and surgical procedures

FVIII coagulation factor VIII, *FIX* coagulation factor IX

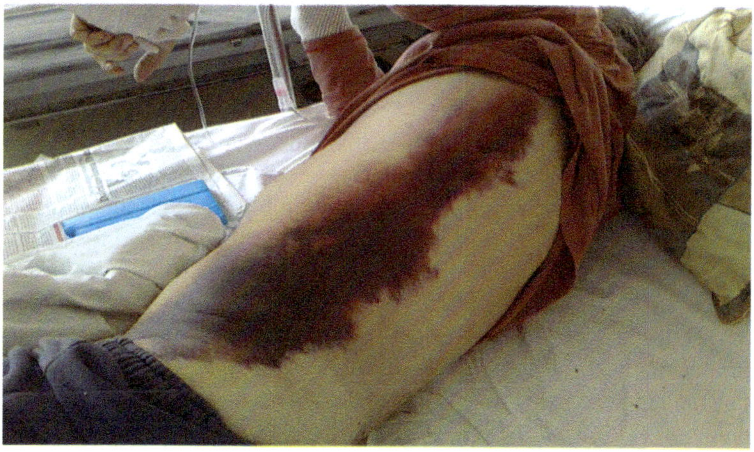

Fig. 12.1 Huge hematoma of the thoracic and abdominal wall in persons with hemophilia

procedures or trauma. The most commonly affected joints are large joints, such as the knee, elbow, and ankle, followed by the shoulder, hip, and wrist. In affected joints, bleeding episodes often recur and are accompanied by pain, swelling, redness, and limited mobility. Such a joint is referred to as a "target joint." Recurrent joint bleeding leads to chronic arthropathy, resulting in deformities, reduced mobility of the affected area, and muscle atrophy. The severe form of the disease typically manifests with bleeding episodes in early childhood, during the period when the child begins to crawl or walk, due to increased physical activity and minor trauma from falls. Intracranial, retroperitoneal or iliopsoas muscle hemorrhages, as well as bleeding in the neck with possible airway obstruction, are critical bleeding sites that pose a life-threatening risk to patients and require urgent treatment [2, 3]. The clinical presentation may also include bleeding from the gastrointestinal tract and hematuria. Bone hemorrhages may result in the formation of pseudotumors, which are predominantly observed in the long bones of the lower extremities. The diagnosis of the mild form of the disease is usually established later in life, given that spontaneous bleeding episodes are rare. The disease typically manifests as prolonged and excessive bleeding following minor procedures in childhood, such as venipuncture, circumcision, deciduous tooth extraction, or severe injuries.

With a better understanding of the disease and advances in treatment, the clinical picture of hemophilia has changed significantly. Early diagnosis of the disease and the prophylactic use of the FVIII clotting factor have significantly reduced the incidence of severe complications and joint-related disability caused by recurrent hemarthroses in the younger population. Furthermore, implementing viral inactivation procedures for plasma-derived clotting factors, along with introducing recombinant factor concentrates, has virtually eliminated the risk of transmitting blood-borne diseases. Today, the life expectancy of persons with mild to moderate hemophilia is approximately equal to that of the general population, while recent therapeutic advances for those with severe forms have significantly contributed not only to increased longevity but also to improved quality of life. The extended life expectancy of persons with hemophilia has drawn greater attention to the management of age-related comorbidities, which, because of the underlying coagulation disorder, require a modified treatment approach.

Although it has long been assumed that women who are carriers of hemophilia with FVIII levels around 50% do not have a tendency toward prolonged bleeding, emerging evidence suggests that some carriers exhibit clinical symptoms consistent with mild hemophilia [1]. Joint bleeding may remain undiagnosed for years, which can lead to serious consequences and poor treatment outcomes for the affected joints. The use of desmopressin (DDAVP) may be particularly important in these persons [1]. If low FVIII levels are detected in carriers, treatment is identical to that used in persons with hemophilia. In female carriers, factor FVIII levels can vary significantly between individuals and may fluctuate considerably during pregnancy and childbirth [2].

Persons with hemophilia A have normal bleeding time (BT), prothrombin time (PT), and thrombin time (TT), while activated partial thromboplastin time (aPTT) is prolonged. Given the low sensitivity and specificity of aPTT, diagnosis is confirmed by demonstrating a reduced FVIII concentration (<40% of normal values) [2, 3, 5]. Genetic testing is performed to confirm the mutation causing the disease, establish the diagnosis in ambiguous cases, assess the risk of inhibitor development, identify female carriers, and support prenatal diagnosis [1, 6].

12.1.1 Treatment of Hemophilia A

In developed countries, the treatment of persons with hemophilia is primarily provided in hemophilia comprehensive care centers (HCCCs). Within these centers, a multidisciplinary team addresses diagnosis, patient education, treatment, and the management of disease- and treatment-related complications. The team includes specialists from various medical disciplines involved in treating this disease, and active patient participation should also be encouraged. The team is led by a hematologist, and a dentist also plays an essential role in the comprehensive care of persons with hemophilia.

The treatment of hemophilia primarily involves factor replacement therapy with clotting factor concentrates (CFC), FVIII for hemophilia A and FIX for hemophilia B. CFC are available as either plasma-derived products, obtained from human donor plasma that has undergone viral inactivation, or as recombinant products, which carry no risk of transmission of blood-borne pathogens. Both recombinant and plasma-derived factor concentrates exhibit comparable efficacy and are considered safe [1].

Recombinant products are indicated for persons who have not been exposed to plasma-derived products and for individuals who are seronegative for HCV and HIV, regardless of prior treatment history [5]. Fresh frozen plasma (FFP) and cryoprecipitate were commonly used to treat hemophilia. These products are less effective than factor concentrates and are currently reserved for situations where specific

CFC are unavailable. In addition to lower efficacy, these products carry a higher risk of transmission of blood-borne infections [1]. Cryoprecipitate contains significant amounts of FVIII, VWF, fibrinogen, and FXIII. One milliliter of FFP is equivalent to 1 international unit (IU) of factor activity [3].

Factor replacement therapy can be administered in both home and hospital settings. Home administration of CFC requires prior patient training. Factor administration can be therapeutic for the management of acute bleeding episodes (episodic or on-demand treatment) or prophylactic, as continuous or intermittent prophylaxis. Prophylactic administration of CFC is used to prevent bleeding, most commonly in children and persons with severe hemophilia. CFC are also administered perioperatively to prevent intra- and postoperative bleeding. On-demand factor treatment helps control bleeding but does not prevent joint damage or long-term complications. When on-demand factor use is indicated, treatment should be initiated as early as possible, as symptoms such as pain often precede objective signs of bleeding. The dose of factor, frequency of administration, and overall duration of therapy depend on the severity of the bleeding episode and the severity of the disease [1, 6].

The biological activity of FVIII concentrate is expressed in IU, where 1 IU/ml of FVIII is equivalent to approximately 200 ng/ml of FVIII in blood. Administration of 1 IU of FVIII per kilogram of body weight is expected to increase plasma FVIII activity by 2% (2 IU/dL) [2–4]. Factor concentrate should be administered 10–20 min before the scheduled surgical procedure to ensure adequate plasma levels at the time of surgery. The following formula is used to calculate the required dose of FVIII [2]:

$$\text{FVIII dose}(\text{IU}) = \text{target FVIII levels} - \text{baseline FVIII levels} \times \text{body weight}(\text{kg}) \times 0.5\,\text{unit} / \text{kg}$$

The half-life of FVIII is approximately 8–12 h. Therefore, it should be administered twice daily to maintain therapeutic levels or, alternatively, via continuous infusion following major surgical procedures. Maximum plasma concentration is achieved 15–30 min after infusion, at which point FVIII levels should be measured to confirm the achieved activity [1]. The target FVIII level depends on the indication for its use. Uncomplicated joint bleeding or superficial hematomas usually require an FVIII level of 30%–50%, whereas larger hematomas or bleeding into deep muscles require an FVIII level > 50%. The duration of therapy depends on the severity and location of bleeding. Life-threatening bleeds, such as oropharyngeal, retroperitoneal, and intracranial hemorrhages, require FVIII levels of 50%–100% maintained over 7–10 days. High-risk surgical procedures may also require high doses of the factor, up to 100% [2, 4, 5]. The length of factor administration after surgery and the applied dose depend on the extent of the procedure and the risk of postoperative bleeding. Perioperative continuous infusion of FVIII concentrate is also a treatment option [1].

Factors are also administered prophylactically to prevent spontaneous bleeding, primarily in the joints. Prophylactic use of FVIII in hemophilia A or FIX in hemophilia B is most often used in persons with severe disease. WFH recommends an individualized approach to prophylactic factor administration for persons with hemophilia A and B with a severe bleeding phenotype [1]. Prophylactic factor administration prevents joint damage, which can lead to reduced mobility and disability. For this reason, this approach is considered significantly superior to on-demand treatment. The purpose of prophylaxis is to enable persons with hemophilia to carry out daily activities without the risk of bleeding. In persons with severe hemophilia, prophylaxis aims to maintain FVIII levels above 1% (usually 3%–5%), effectively converting severe to moderate hemophilia and reducing the risk of spontaneous bleeding [1]. Prophylactic administration of coagulation factors can be classified as primary, secondary, or tertiary. Primary prophylaxis refers to the administration of coagulation factor before the onset of joint damage, before the second clinically evident joint bleed, and before age 3. This type of prophylaxis is considered the most effective for preventing the development of hemophilic arthropathy. Secondary prophylaxis refers to the administration of factors after two or more clinically evident joint bleeds, when joint damage has not yet occurred, usually after age 3. Tertiary prophylaxis aims to prevent further disease progression in cases where joint damage has already occurred and is typically implemented in adulthood [1, 3]. FVIII is administered prophylactically two to three times per week, while FIX is given twice a week. The intensity of prophylaxis refers to both the dose and frequency of factor administration and can be classified as high-, intermediate-, and low-dose prophylaxis. Fixed prophylactic regimens for hemophilia A and hemophilia B with standard half-life factors involve administration of: FVIII 25–40 IU/kg per dose every 2 days or FIX 40–60 IU/kg per dose twice a week (high-dose prophylaxis); FVIII 15–25 IU/kg 3 days a week or FIX 20–40 IU/kg twice a week (intermediate-dose prophylaxis); and FVIII 10–15 IU/kg 2–3 days a week or FIX 10–15 IU/kg twice a week (low-dose prophylaxis) [1]. In addition to fixed prophylactic regimens, an individualized approach based on disease severity and the bleeding phenotype is also used. With the introduction of new therapeutic modalities for the treatment of hemophilia, the modern definition of prophylaxis includes not only regular prophylactic intravenous administration of CFC but also continuous use of other therapeutic agents to prevent bleeding in persons with hemophilia. This enables persons with hemophilia to engage in regular daily activities and ensures a quality of life similar to that of the non-hemophilic population [1].

In recent years, long-acting factor products and alternative therapies (e.g., emicizumab for hemophilia A, with or without inhibitors) have been developed. The use of these agents reduces the need for frequent infusions. These new therapies have significantly changed the prophylactic approach in persons with hemophilia, allowing higher, more stable factor levels to be maintained for longer periods.

12.1.2 Complications of Transfusion Therapy in Hemophilia A

Historically, the primary complication of frequent blood transfusions and blood products was the risk of transmitting blood-borne infections, including hepatitis B, hepatitis C, and human immunodeficiency virus (HIV). The introduction of viral inactivation procedures for plasma-derived products in the mid-1980s significantly reduced the risk of transmission of these infections. However, a theoretical risk of transmission of both known and unknown infectious agents remains, including parvovirus B19 and prion diseases (e.g., Creutzfeldt-Jakob disease). With the introduction of recombinant coagulation factors into clinical practice in the 1990s, this risk was eliminated. The use of the hepatitis B vaccine further reduces the risk of transmission of this virus. In persons with hemophilia who are infected with hepatitis B or C virus, potential liver dysfunction should be considered during treatment or surgical preparation. Additionally, individuals with HIV infection may be immunocompromised.

The development of autoantibodies (inhibitors) against FVIII or FIX is currently considered the most common complication of transfusion therapy in hemophilia. Inhibitors are IgG-class immunoglobulins that neutralize therapeutic FVIII or FIX. Inhibitors are estimated to develop in approximately 30% of persons with severe hemophilia A and in about 5%–10% of those with mild or moderate hemophilia A. The cumulative incidence of inhibitor development in persons with hemophilia B is up to 5% [1–4]. Inhibitors can develop following the administration of both plasma-derived and recombinant FVIII or FIX concentrates, typically after the first 20 exposures [1, 6]. The underlying mechanism of inhibitor development involves an immune response, but the precise immunological mechanism remains unclear. Factors contributing to inhibitor development may be person-related or treatment-related. There is a higher predisposition for inhibitor development in persons with the severe form of the disease, a family history of inhibitors, severe genetic mutations, of Black African descent, and high-intensity factor exposure (high doses, more frequently, for a longer period, and at an earlier age) [1, 3, 6]. The development of inhibitors presents a greater clinical challenge due to the increased risk of bleeding and the complexities of treatment.

Inhibitors are suspected when there is an inadequate clinical or laboratory response to administered FVIII or FIX concentrate, despite prior effective treatment. Routine inhibitor screening is recommended, initially every 6–12 months after a newly diagnosed case of hemophilia and initiation of CFC treatment, and subsequently annually thereafter [1]. Inhibitor screening should also be performed after initial exposure to coagulation factors, in persons with frequent joint bleeding despite CFC administration, following prolonged use of factor replacement therapy (typically over 5 consecutive days), in persons who do not respond adequately to factor replacement therapy, and prior to major surgical procedures [1]. In persons with hemophilia who do not have inhibitors, the aPTT is corrected by adding normal plasma to the patient's plasma in a 1:1 ratio. In persons with inhibitors, the aPTT remains prolonged after the addition of normal plasma (1:1) because of the presence of inhibitors and the resulting neutralization of FVIII. Inhibitors are detected and quantified by the Bethesda or Nijmegen-modified Bethesda assay. Bethesda units (BU) are used to quantify and express the antibody titer. The presence of inhibitors is confirmed when the antibody titer is 0.6 BU/mL for FVIII and ≥0.3 BU/mL for FIX. A low inhibitor titer is defined as <5.0 BU/mL, whereas a high titer is ≥5.0 BU/mL [1]. Persons with a low antibody titer (<5 BU/mL) generally have a weak response to the administered CFC, which does not significantly reduce treatment effectiveness (low-responding inhibitors). A rapid and strong reaction to factor replacement therapy is usually observed in patients with high antibody titers ≥5.0 BU/mL (high-responding inhibitors). In cases of low inhibitor titer, antibody levels tend to decline over time, usually within 6 months, regardless of CFC administration. In persons with a high inhibitor titer, the high titer persists for a long time and decreases only when there is no exposure to CFC. However, re-exposure to CFC increases the inhibitor titer for 3–5 days after factor administration [1].

The treatment of a person with hemophilia and inhibitors can be divided into two goals: stopping bleeding and eradicating the inhibitors. In persons with low-responding inhibitors who develop an acute bleed, high doses of CFC replacement therapy are recommended. For high-responding inhibitors, bypassing agents such as activated prothrombin complex concentrate (aPCC) or activated recombinant FVII (rFVIIa) are used in case of acute bleeding [1, 2, 6]. Both bypassing agents have comparable efficacy. However, in specific clinical situations, one may be more effective than the other. For joint bleeding episodes, treatment commonly involves the administration of two doses of rFVIIa (90–270 μg/kg) or one dose of aPCC (75–85 units/kg) [1]. These two agents can also be administered in combination. rFVIIa binds to tissue factor, leading to the activation of factors X and IX, thus facilitating the progression of the coagulation cascade. aPCC contains non-activated FII, FIX, and FX, as well as activated FVII. It is used in persons with hemophilia A, hemophilia B, and inhibitors. In persons with hemophilia B and inhibitors who exhibit an allergic reaction to FIX, the aPCC should not be used, as it may trigger an allergic reaction [1]. Both bypassing agents are also used for bleeding prevention prior to surgical procedures.

Eradication of inhibitors by immune tolerance induction (ITI) requires frequent, usually daily, administration of the missing factor and lasts for several months, sometimes longer than a year. Dose and frequency of factor administration may vary. The success rate of ITI is approximately 70%–80% in persons with severe hemophilia A [1, 2, 6]. ITI is less successful in persons with a mild or moderate form of the disease. ITI is considered unsuccessful if a high inhibitor titer persists and there is no clinical response to FVIII replacement therapy within 2–3 years of initiating ITI [1].

In persons refractory to ITI, an anti-CD20 monoclonal antibody (rituximab) may be administered in conjunction with ITI [2]. In cases of ITI failure, prophylaxis with emicizumab is recommended [1]. Because of the lower incidence of inhibitor development in persons with hemophilia B, ITI has not been adequately evaluated in clinical studies. An additional challenge is the potential for allergic reactions to the administered FIX [6].

Emicizumab, a monoclonal antibody, is used for the prophylaxis of bleeding in persons with hemophilia A, both with and without inhibitors. For persons with hemophilia A and low-titer inhibitors receiving emicizumab prophylaxis, FVIII replacement therapy is recommended in the event of a bleeding episode [1]. For persons with hemophilia A and high-titer inhibitors, rFVIIa should be preferred over aPCC to avoid the risk of thrombotic microangiopathy [1].

12.1.3 Non-transfusion Therapy in Hemophilia A

Non-transfusion management of hemophilia A involves the administration of DDAVP, antifibrinolytic agents and the use of new innovative therapies (see Sect. 12.1.4). DDAVP is a synthetic analog of the antidiuretic hormone vasopressin. It transiently increases plasma FVIII and VWF, promoting their release from endothelial cells. Released VWF binds to FVIII, stabilizing it in circulation. DDAVP is used only in persons with mild or moderate hemophilia A, for whom its clinical efficacy has been previously confirmed. It can be administered intravenously, subcutaneously, or as a nasal spray. Intravenous DDAVP infusion over 20–30 min at a dose of 0.3 μg/kg body weight induces a three- to sixfold increase in FVIII levels relative to baseline, with a peak occurring approximately 60 min after infusion [1, 2, 6]. The half-life of released FVIII is 8–12 h. A repeated dose of DDAVP is less effective due to depletion of FVIII and VWF stores. It is administered 12 h after the initial dose, with the possibility of one additional dose thereafter. This phenomenon is called tachyphylaxis. After three repeated doses, further treatment is usually ineffective and requires the administration of CFC [2]. The use of DDAVP is not recommended for more than three consecutive days [1]. The dose of DDAVP for subcutaneous administration is 0.3 μg/kg, up to a maximum of 15 μg. Intranasal DDAVP is administered at a dose of 300 μg (1.5 mg/mL in each nostril) in patients weighing more than 50 kg and 150 μg (1.5 mg/mL in a single nostril) in patients weighing less than 50 kg [1]. Intranasal DDAVP may be less effective than subcutaneous use. Given that DDAVP is an antidiuretic, the most serious adverse effect is water retention, which may lead to hyponatremia. Other side effects include headache, flushing, tremor, weakness, tachycardia, and abdominal pain [1]. DDAVP is not effective in persons with severe forms of hemophilia A, as well as in persons with hemophilia B.

Antifibrinolytics (tranexamic acid, TA, and ε-aminocaproic acid, EACA) are effective in controlling mucosal bleeding, such as gingival bleeding, epistaxis, menorrhagia, gastrointestinal bleeding, and bleeding following oral surgical procedures. These agents prevent the activation of plasminogen to plasmin. TA is administered orally at a dose of 25 mg/kg, three to four times daily. Treatment usually lasts for 7 days. It can also be administered intravenously at a dose of 10 mg/kg, two to three times daily [1, 2, 7]. EACA is less commonly used due to shorter half-life, lower efficacy, and higher toxicity compared to TA. EACA is administered orally at a dose of 100 mg/kg (up to a maximum of 2 g per dose) or intravenously at a dose of 100 mg/kg (up to maximum of 4 g per dose) every 4–6 h. The maximum dose is 24 g per day [1, 2]. For the prevention of postoperative bleeding, antifibrinolytic therapy should be initiated before the surgical intervention. For intraoral bleeding, antifibrinolytics can also be used locally in the form of mouthwash solutions. TA is used as a 5% mouthwash solution at a dose of 10 mL, four times a day, for 7 days following dental procedures [7]. Antifibrinolytics can be used alone, with CFC or bypassing agents. The main side effect of antifibrinolytic use is gastrointestinal discomfort.

12.1.4 New Therapies for Hemophilia

New treatment approaches for persons with hemophilia include extended half-life factors, nonfactor replacement therapy, drugs that inhibit natural anticoagulants, and gene therapy.

The requirement for frequent administration of CFC for prophylaxis imposes a significant treatment burden on persons with hemophilia. The introduction of extended half-life clotting factors into clinical practice reduces the need for frequent CFC administration and improves quality of life for persons with hemophilia. Extended half-life clotting factors are produced using advanced biotechnological methods, including PEGylation or fusion to albumin or immunoglobulin [1, 6].

Extended half-life FVIII products have a 1.4- to 1.6-fold longer half-life than standard FVIII products and are administered twice a week for prophylaxis in persons with hemophilia. Extended half-life FIX products are administered once a week or once every 2 weeks, with a duration three to five times longer than that of standard FIX CFC [1, 2, 6].

Emicizumab (ACE910) is a recombinant bispecific monoclonal antibody that binds to FIXa and FX, replacing the function of missing FVIIIa in the coagulation process. Unlike traditional treatment for hemophilia, which involves replacing the missing clotting factor, emicizumab mimics the function of FVIII and acts as a substitute for the deficient FVIII. It has been in clinical use since 2018 and is gradually becoming the standard of care for persons with severe hemophilia A, with or without inhibitors [1, 8]. It is administered subcutaneously, once a week or once every 2 or 4 weeks, significantly reducing the frequency of bleeding complications in persons with hemophilia A, regardless of inhibitor status [1, 9–13]. The recommended dose is 3 mg/kg once weekly for the first 4 weeks (loading dose), followed by a maintenance dose starting in week 5 of either 1.5 mg/kg once weekly, 3 mg/kg every 2 weeks, or 6 mg/kg every 4 weeks [1, 8]. The drug is administered prophylactically and is not indicated for the management of acute hemorrhagic events. For persons who develop an acute bleed while receiving emicizumab prophylaxis, either FVIII CFC or rFVIIa is used, depending on the severity of bleeding and the presence of inhibitors. Emicizumab prophylaxis has led to a substantial shift in the therapeutic management of hemophilia, effectively converting severe hemophilia into a mild form. The subcutaneous route of administration offers a considerable advantage compared to intravenous infusion of CFC. The primary adverse reaction associated with the drug is an injection site reaction, which is typically mild [13].

Inhibitors of natural anticoagulants (antithrombin inhibitors and tissue factor pathway inhibitors, anti-TFPI) are also referred to as hemostatic rebalancing agents. Fitusiran acts by suppressing hepatic production of antithrombin. It has a prolonged effect, is administered subcutaneously, and could be used in persons with hemophilia A and B, with or without inhibitors [1]. Marstacimab and concizumab are monoclonal antibodies that inhibit TFPI, thereby increasing thrombin levels and facilitating the coagulation process. These drugs were recently approved for clinical use in some countries, but there remains a need for long-term observation of persons receiving these drugs, and questions remain regarding the monitoring of hemostatic function as well as the evaluation of potential thrombotic risk [14, 15].

Gene therapy for hemophilia has recently been introduced into clinical practice as a one-time treatment for persons with hemophilia A and hemophilia B [16, 17]. Gene therapy involves a single intravenous administration of a recombinant adeno-associated virus serotype 5 (AAV5) vector that delivers a functional gene to replace the patient's defective gene, thereby restoring liver production of the deficient coagulation factor. One reason for limited use of gene therapy for hemophilia is the high price and uncertainty of reimbursement by national health care systems.

12.2 Hemophilia B

Hemophilia B (Christmas disease) is an inherited coagulopathy caused by a deficiency of FIX. The disorder is inherited in an X-linked recessive pattern and results from mutations in the *F9* gene, which encodes FIX. The estimated prevalence at birth is 5 cases per 100,000 males, of which 1.5 cases are the severe form of the disease [1]. The severe form of the disease is defined by a FIX level of less than 1% and is characterized by spontaneous bleeding. The moderate and mild forms of the disease are defined by FIX levels between 1%–5% and above 5%, respectively (Table 12.1). In general, the clinical manifestations of hemophilia B are similar to those of hemophilia A; however, severe forms of the disease are less common. Persons with hemophilia B have a prolonged aPTT, and the definitive diagnosis is established by confirming reduced FIX levels.

Treatment of hemophilia B primarily involves administering FIX CFC, which may be human plasma-derived or recombinant. aPCC, which contains factors II, VII, IX, and X, is rarely used to treat hemophilia B because of the risk of thromboembolism. FIX replacement therapy can be used to treat acute bleeding or as prophylaxis (see Sect. 12.1.1). One unit (IU) of FIX CFC corresponds to the amount of FIX present in 1 mL of normal plasma (5 μg/mL) [2]. One IU of FIX per kilogram of body weight raises the FIX concentration by approximately 1% (1 IU/dL) [2–4]. The formula for FIX replacement differs from that used for FVIII replacement [2]:

$$\text{FIX dose}(\text{IU}) = \text{target FIX levels} - \text{baseline FIX levels} \times \text{body weight}(\text{kg}) \times 1\,\text{unit}/\text{kg}$$

The half-life of FIX is longer than that of FVIII, approximately 18–24 h, so a single FIX CFC infusion per day is usually sufficient. The achieved FIX level in circulation should be tested 15–30 min after CFC infusion [1]. DDAVP is not used in the treatment of hemophilia B because it has no effect on FIX concentration in plasma.

In case of inhibitor development, the treatment (similar to the one used in persons with hemophilia A and inhibitors) is applied. In persons with low-responding inhibitors (<5 BU/ml), who develop an acute bleed, high-doses of FIX replacement therapy is recommended with caution, including monitoring of potential allergic reactions. For high-responding inhibitors (≥5,0 BU/ml), bypassing agents, such as aPCC or rFVIIa, are used in case of acute bleeding. In a case of allergic reaction to FIX, rFVIIa is used, as aPCC may trigger an allergic response [1].

12.3 Deficiency of Coagulation Factor XI and Rare Coagulopathies

Activated FXI (FXIa) participates in the intrinsic coagulation pathway by catalyzing FIX activation. FXI activation is mediated by FXIIa in the presence of high-molecular-weight kininogen (HMWK) and kallikrein. In vivo, FXI is also activated by thrombin [2]. Patients with FXI deficiency cannot activate thrombin-activatable fibrinolysis inhibitor (TAFI), resulting in accelerated fibrinolysis.

FXI deficiency is a rare bleeding disorder affecting approximately one in a million people [2]. The normal range of FXI coagulant activity is 70–150 U/dL. Patients with FXI levels below 20 U/dL have a severe bleeding disorder [4], and levels below 10% of normal are typically associated with a high risk of bleeding [2]. However, the severity of the clinical presentation, or bleeding phenotype, does not always correlate with the plasma concentration of FXI [2]. The disorder is inherited in an autosomal recessive manner and clinically manifests as mucocutaneous bleeding, gingival bleeding, epistaxis, hematuria, menorrhagia, and bleeding following trauma and surgical interventions. Unlike hemophilia, spontaneous bleeding into joints and muscles is not typical. Treatment involves administration of FFP, FXI concentrates, and antifibrinolytic agents [2, 4]. Development of inhibitors against FXI is possible, and in such cases, aPCC or rFVIIa may be used for acute bleeding [2, 4].

The term "rare coagulopathies" refers to congenital deficiencies of any of the coagulation factors, excluding FVIII, FIX, and FXI. Deficiencies of fibrinogen, prothrombin, FV, FVII, FX, FXII, FXIII, HMWK, and kallikrein have been described. These disorders are inherited in an autosomal recessive manner. Clinical presentation ranges from asymptomatic forms to life-threatening conditions. When symptoms are present, mucocutaneous bleeding usually predominates, whereas bleeding into joints is rare. The clinical presentation does not indicate a deficiency of a specific factor. The disorder is diagnosed using routine laboratory tests to evaluate hemostasis, followed by confirmation of a specific factor deficiency. Treatment involves the use of FFP and aPCC. CFC are available for FVII and FXIII deficiency [2, 4, 18]. Unlike other clotting factor deficiencies, factor XII deficiency is completely asymptomatic and does not cause excess bleeding even after major surgical procedures or trauma. Associations between FXII deficiency and spontaneous abortion, premature delivery, arterial and venous thromboses, myocardial infarction, and PE have been reported. FXII also plays an important role in inflammation, sepsis, and hereditary angioedema [19].

In addition to single-factor deficiencies, combined deficiencies of several coagulation factors have also been described. These disorders are very rare, and patients usually have a positive family history. Among these disorders, combined FV and

FVIII deficiency and multiple deficiencies of vitamin K-dependent coagulation factors stand out. The latter is caused by mutations in genes responsible for synthesizing enzymes involved in vitamin K metabolism (γ-glutamylcarboxylase and epoxide reductase) [2].

Recommendations for the dental management of patients with rare coagulopathies are similar to those for persons with hemophilia. In cases of severe disease and extensive oral surgical procedures, preoperative use of coagulation factors is required.

References

1. Srivastava A, Santagostino E, Dougall A, Kitchen S, Sutherland M, Pipe SW, Carcao M, Mahlangu J, Ragni MV, Windyga J, Llinás A, Goddard NJ, Mohan R, Poonnoose PM, Feldman BM, Lewis SZ, van den Berg HM, Pierce GF, WFH Guidelines for the Management of Hemophilia Panelists, et al. WFH guidelines for the management of hemophilia, 3rd edition. Haemophilia. 2020;26(Suppl 6):1–158. Erratum in: Haemophilia 2021;27(4):699.
2. Arruda VR, High KA. Coagulation disorders. In: Harrison's principles of internal medicine. 20th ed. McGraw-Hill Education eBook; 2018. p. 830–8.
3. Gangwani P, Richards R. Review of hemophilia A and B and perioperative management in dentistry. In: Szumita RP, Szumita PM, editors. Hemostasis in dentistry. Springer; 2018. p. 33–8.
4. Bermudez P, Beushausen M, Horan MP. Management of inherited, acquired, and iatrogenically induced coagulopathies in oral surgery. In: A textbook of advanced oral and maxillofacial surgery, vol. 3. InTech; 2016. p. 175–210.
5. Little JW, Miller CS, Rhodus NL. Congenital bleeding and hypercoagulable disorders. In: Little and Falace's dental management of the medically compromised patient. 9th ed. St. Louis: Elsevier; 2018. p. 457–79.
6. Peyvandi F, Garagiola I, Young G. The past and future of haemophilia: diagnosis, treatments, and its complications. Lancet. 2016;388(10040):187–97.
7. Scully C. Haemathology. In: Scully's medical problems in dentistry. 7th ed. Elsevier: Churchill Livingstone; 2014. p. 212–75.
8. Mahlangu J, Iorio A, Kenet G. Emicizumab state-of-the-art update. Haemophilia. 2022;28(Suppl 4):103–10.
9. Oldenburg J, Mahlangu JN, Kim B, Schmitt C, Callaghan MU, Young G, Santagostino E, Kruse-Jarres R, Negrier C, Kessler C, Valente N, Asikanius E, Levy GG, Windyga J, Shima M. Emicizumab prophylaxis in hemophilia A with inhibitors. N Engl J Med. 2017;377(9):809–18.
10. Young G, Liesner R, Chang T, Sidonio R, Oldenburg J, Jiménez-Yuste V, Mahlangu J, Kruse-Jarres R, Wang M, Uguen M, Doral MY, Wright LY, Schmitt C, Levy GG, Shima M, Mancuso ME. A multicenter, open-label phase 3 study of emicizumab prophylaxis in children with hemophilia A with inhibitors. Blood. 2019;134(24):2127–38.
11. Mahlangu J, Oldenburg J, Paz-Priel I, Negrier C, Niggli M, Mancuso ME, Schmitt C, Jiménez-Yuste V, Kempton C, Dhalluin C, Callaghan MU, Bujan W, Shima M, Adamkewicz JI, Asikanius E, Levy GG, Kruse-Jarres R. Emicizumab prophylaxis in patients who have hemophilia A without inhibitors. N Engl J Med. 2018;379(9):811–22.
12. Pipe SW, Shima M, Lehle M, Shapiro A, Chebon S, Fukutake K, Key NS, Portron A, Schmitt C, Podolak-Dawidziak M, Selak Bienz N, Hermans C, Campinha-Bacote A, Kiialainen A, Peerlinck K, Levy GG, Jiménez-Yuste V. Efficacy, safety, and pharmacokinetics of emicizumab prophylaxis given every 4 weeks in people with haemophilia A (HAVEN 4): a multicentre, open-label, non-randomised phase 3 study. Lancet Haematol. 2019;6(6):e295–305.

13. Callaghan MU, Negrier C, Paz-Priel I, Chang T, Chebon S, Lehle M, Mahlangu J, Young G, Kruse-Jarres R, Mancuso ME, Niggli M, Howard M, Bienz NS, Shima M, Jiménez-Yuste V, Schmitt C, Asikanius E, Levy GG, Pipe SW, Oldenburg J. Long-term outcomes with emicizumab prophylaxis for hemophilia A with or without FVIII inhibitors from the HAVEN 1–4 studies. Blood. 2021;137(16):2231–42.
14. Mancuso ME, Croteau SE, Klamroth R. Benefits and risks of non-factor therapies: redefining haemophilia treatment goals in the era of new technologies. Haemophilia. 2024;30(Suppl 3):39–44.
15. Jiménez-Yuste V. Non-factor therapies for hemophilia: achievements and perspectives. Semin Thromb Hemost. 2025;51(1):23–7.
16. Leavitt AD, Mahlangu J, Raheja P, Symington E, Quon DV, Giermasz A, López Fernández MF, Kenet G, Lowe G, Key NS, Millar CM, Pipe SW, Madan B, Chou SC, Klamroth R, Mason J, Chambost H, Peyvandi F, Majerus E, Pepperell D, Rivat C, Yu H, Robinson TM, Ozelo MC. Efficacy, safety, and quality of life 4 years after valoctocogene roxaparvovec gene transfer for severe hemophilia A in the phase 3 GENEr8-1 trial. Res Pract Thromb Haemost. 2024;8(8):102615.
17. von Drygalski A, Gomez E, Giermasz A, Castaman G, Key NS, Lattimore SU, Leebeek FWG, Miesbach WA, Recht M, Monahan PE, Le Quellec S, Pipe SW. Completion of phase 2b trial of etranacogene dezaparvovec gene therapy in patients with hemophilia B over 5 years. Blood Adv. 2025;9(14):3543–52.
18. Israels S, Schwetz N, Boyar R, McNicol A. Bleeding disorders: characterization, dental considerations and management. J Can Dent Assoc. 2006;72(9):827.
19. Maas C, Renne T. Coagulation factor XII in thrombosis and inflammation. Blood. 2018;131(17):1903–9.

Dental Management of Persons with Hemophilia

13

Branislav V. Bajkin and Alison Dougall

Box 13.1 Dental Considerations in PwH

1. *Hemophilia A (FVIII deficiency)*
2. *Hemophilia B (FIX deficiency)*
   - *Severity of the disease*
     - *Severe (FVIII/FIX <1% of normal)*
     - *Moderate (FVIII/FIX 1%–5% of normal)*
     - *Mild (FVIII/FIX 5%–40% of normal)*

High importance of prevention of oral diseases

- Gingival bleeding is more related to poor oral hygiene and local inflammation than to the disease itself

Oral surgery in PwH

- Consult the patient's physician
- Individualized dental treatment plan in discussion with a hematologist
- Decision on Inpatient or outpatient treatment depending on the bleeding risk of the procedure
- Perioperative hematological treatment* depends on the risk of the procedure, type and the severity of the disease and may include DDAVP, FVIII, or FIX concentrate and antifibrinolytics

(continued)

B. V. Bajkin (✉)
University of Novi Sad, Faculty of Medicine, Dentistry Clinic of Vojvodina, Novi Sad, Serbia
e-mail: branislav.bajkin@mf.uns.ac.rs

A. Dougall
School of Dental Science, Trinity College Dublin, Dublin Dental University Hospital, Dublin, Ireland

B. V. Bajkin (ed.), *Bleeding Disorders and Dentistry*,
https://doi.org/10.1007/978-3-032-26713-9_13

Box 13.1 (continued)

  - DDAVP may be effective in mild and in some moderate forms of hemophilia A
  - DDAVP responsiveness should be obtained before using DDAVP for therapeutic interventions
  - FVIII concentrate should be used in PwH A with severe form of the disease and in other forms in PwH A with lack of DDAVP efficacy
  - FIX concentrate should be used in PwH B
  - Use of antifibrinolytics systemically and/or locally along with DDAVP and FVIII or FIX concentrate
- Be aware of possible life-threatening bleeding in the floor of the mouth
- Schedule a patient at the beginning of the work week
- Use of local anesthesia with vasoconstrictor
- IANB and lingual infiltration anesthesia require factor replacement
- Consider alternative local anesthetic techniques to avoid IANB (see Table 13.1)
- Minimally traumatic surgical technique
- Use of local hemostatic agents and measures to control oral bleeding
- Local use of antifibrinolytics in the form of mouthwash solution may be of great importance
- For pain relief use acetaminophen or selective C0X-2 inhibitors; avoid aspirin and other NSAIDs
- Provide a patient with postoperative instructions (soft and cold diet, phone number in case of an emergency) and regular follow-up

F VIII coagulation factor VIII, *FIX* coagulation factor IX, *PwH* person with hemophilia A or B, *DDAVP* desmopressin, *IANB* inferior alveolar nerve block, *COX-2* cyclooxigenase-2, *NSAIDs* nonsteroidal anti-inflammatory drugs

*Proposed hematological treatments vary from pre- and postoperative factor replacement and single-dose preoperative factor replacement to no factor replacement. Recent studies mostly support single-dose preoperative factor replacement to achieve factor plasma levels of 30%–50% along with the use of antifibrinolytics [1]

Table 13.1 Local anesthesia in persons with hemophilia

Clotting factor replacement required	Alternative techniques for IANB that do not require clotting factor replacement
Inferior alveolar nerve block (IANB)	Posterior mandible 4% articaine mandibular buccal infiltration
Other "block" techniques with high bleeding risk (e.g. posterior superior alveolar nerve block)	Anterior mandible Mental nerve block without needle insertion into the foramen Buccal infiltration for incisors
Lingual infiltration	Intraligamentary injection Single tooth anesthesia applied with computer-controlled local anaesthetic delivery system

For many years, myths and dogmas have suggested that every dental procedure in persons with hemophilia requires factor replacement therapy. Newer evidence-based recommendations suggest the opposite; the majority of dental procedures in persons with hemophilia can be performed with minimal use of clotting factor concentrates (CFC) or without them. This chapter presents the dental aspects of hemophilia A and hemophilia B together, considering the similarities in clinical manifestations of these diseases, the risk of postoperative bleeding, and the similarities in perioperative treatment.

For all patients with bleeding disorders, maintaining oral and dental health and preventing bleeding after dental procedures are of utmost importance. A thorough medical history can reveal prior spontaneous bleeding episodes and bleeding after trauma or surgical procedures, including tooth extractions. Because these are inherited coagulation disorders, a positive family history is usually present. Clinical examination may reveal skin hematomas, pain, swelling, and limited mobility of the affected ("target") joints.

Prevention of oral diseases should begin as early as possible, ideally at the eruption of the first primary tooth, typically between 6 months and 1 year of age [2].

Immediately after a hemophilia diagnosis, parents should receive comprehensive information on the importance of optimal oral hygiene. Preventive dental measures and regular dental checkups should be integrated into the comprehensive care program for persons with hemophilia. Preventive measures include preventive dental visits, adherence to dietary advice with a reduction in carbohydrate intake, motivation and training in proper oral hygiene, local fluoride application, and fissure sealing. It is recommended to brush teeth and the mouth at least twice a day using soft- or medium-bristle toothbrushes and fluoride-containing toothpaste. The use of topical fluoride preparations, such as gels, mouth rinses, and tablets, should be adjusted based on the fluoride concentration in the drinking water. Additional measures (the use of dental floss, interdental brushes, antibacterial mouthwash solutions, and water-jet devices) are recommended for proper oral hygiene and the prevention of caries and periodontal diseases on approximal tooth surfaces. Intake of foods and beverages with high sugar content should be limited to mealtimes, and the use of artificial sweeteners is also recommended. Regular dental checkups should be scheduled every 6 months [2–4]. Prevention of oral and dental diseases in childhood reduces the need for invasive dental procedures later in life and significantly contributes to quality of life in persons with inherited bleeding disorders [2, 5].

Results from studies of oral health status in persons with inherited coagulopathies are inconsistent. Some studies in children [6–10] and adults [11] reported higher dmf-t/DMF-T (decayed, missing, and filled teeth) indices in persons with hemophilia and von Willebrand disease (VWD) compared with a control group without these diseases. In contrast, the majority of recent studies do not indicate poorer oral health in children [12–16] and adults [17] with inherited coagulopathies compared with persons without these diseases. In addition, some studies have shown that oral health in children with hemophilia is better than in a control group of healthy participants [18–22]. Furthermore, some studies reported better oral health in persons with severe hemophilia than in those with a mild form of the disease [5]. These contradictory research results are more likely associated with the availability of dental care services and the development of preventive dental programs in the countries where such studies were conducted, as well as with the personal motivation of patients, children, and their parents, rather than with the disease itself [23].

During dental procedures, extra care is required to avoid accidental injury to the soft tissues of the oral cavity. Examples include the use of suction devices, removal of cotton rolls, placement of matrix bands and wooden wedges, impression taking for prosthodontic or orthodontic treatment, and the placement of intraoral films or plates during intraoral radiography, all of which may result in accidental injury and necessitate additional caution.

It is well established that most dental procedures do not require preoperative administration of factor replacement. Furthermore, most procedures, including many in oral surgery, can be safely performed in outpatient settings without hospitalization. Dental procedures that do not require factor replacement include restorative procedures, root canal treatment, removable prosthodontics, fixed and removable orthodontic appliances, and supragingival scaling [3, 24–26]. During endodontic treatment, it is essential to carefully determine the working length of the root canal and avoid irritation of the periapical tissues.

Periodontal procedures require a cautious approach because of tissue manipulation and the potential for increased bleeding. Achieving local hemostasis in cases of gingival bleeding can be challenging. In cases of severe gingival inflammation, the inflammation should be managed first by supragingival scaling, motivation and instruction in proper oral hygiene measures, rinsing the mouth with antibacterial solutions, and, if needed, antibiotic therapy. Supragingival scaling can be safely performed without factor replacement therapy, whereas subgingival scaling should be performed with great caution and only after the inflammation has decreased. It is recommended that treatment be carried out over multiple visits to minimize the risk of excessive and prolonged bleeding. The use of lasers during periodontal procedures can be highly important, particularly for achieving hemostasis and reducing the bacterial load [27]. Periodontal surgical procedures are considered high risk and require adequate preoperative management with coagulation factor replacement therapy [3, 24, 25]. In contrast to post-extraction wounds, where local hemostatic agents can be easily applied, their effectiveness is often limited in cases of extensive gingival bleeding because of the larger bleeding surface. Nonetheless, the importance of antifibrinolytics in managing mucosal bleeding within the oral cavity should be emphasized. Antifibrinolytics can be used systemically or locally, either directly applied to the wound or as a mouthwash solution.

13.1 Local Anesthesia and Pain Management in Persons with Hemophilia

The majority of dental interventions require local anesthesia to ensure adequate pain control and patient comfort. No local anesthetic agent has an absolute advantage over others. However, given the benefits of local hemostasis and the intensity and duration of the anesthetic effect, the use of a local anesthetic with a vasoconstrictor is recommended in persons with bleeding disorders. Slow administration of the local anesthetic, along with the use of needles with a smaller gauge (Fig. 1.3), reduces tissue trauma at the injection site. Additional safety can be achieved through the use of computer-controlled local anesthetic delivery devices.

Certain local anesthesia techniques, such as buccal infiltration, intraligamentary and intrapapillary injections, and mental nerve block without inserting the needle into the mental foramen, are considered safe in persons with hemophilia without factor replacement. These techniques are always preferred over block anesthesia techniques, such as the inferior alveolar nerve block (IANB) and the posterior superior alveolar nerve block, which require factor replacement because of the risk of bleeding [3, 24].

Bleeding into the loose connective tissue of the floor of the oral cavity within a short period can lead to airway obstruction. Therefore, infiltration of local anesthesia into the floor of the oral cavity in persons with hemophilia requires factor replacement therapy. During IANB, the needle enters the pterygomandibular space by penetrating the medial pterygoid muscle. Bleeding within the muscle and the pterygomandibular space can also lead to airway obstruction; therefore, this anesthesia technique requires hemostatic cover with the deficient coagulation factor [3, 4, 24]. There is some evidence that in persons with mild hemophilia or those on continuous factor prophylaxis, the IANB can be performed successfully without factor replacement [28]. One factor contributing to the safety of this anesthesia technique is the use of currently available cartridge syringes and needles with significantly smaller diameters, which reduce tissue trauma [25]. However, this approach is not widely accepted, and further research is needed to confirm its safety.

Anesthesia of mandibular posterior teeth is usually achieved by IANB. When performing tooth extraction in persons with hemophilia, IANB generally does not pose a problem, provided the procedure is carried out with factor replacement therapy. However, for restorative or endodontic procedures in this region, the question arises whether there is an adequate alternative to IANB that would not require the use of CFC. Intraligamentary anesthesia and buccal infiltration of anesthetic into the mandibular vestibule are alternative techniques that do not require factor replacement therapy (Table 13.1). Numerous studies have demonstrated that buccal infiltration of 4% articaine provides satisfactory pulpal anesthesia in mandibular posterior teeth [29, 30]. The high success rate and safety of buccal infiltration with 4% articaine with adrenaline 1:100,000 and 2% lignocaine with adrenaline 1:80,000 have been confirmed for various dental procedures, such as fillings, root canal, and scaling, in persons with mild, moderate, and severe hemophilia without CFC cover [31]. In recent years, computer-controlled local anesthetic delivery has been introduced, enabling single-tooth anesthesia via an intraligamentary injection. Computer-controlled injection systems provide continuous, slow application of anesthetic, making the procedure less painful. An additional benefit of these devices is their integrated self-aspiration capability, which enhances safety during anesthetic administration. Single-tooth anesthesia appears to be an extremely suitable technique for persons with hemophilia, in whom the use of IANB and hemostatic cover with CFC is to be avoided [27].

Management of pain associated with oral and dental pathology should focus primarily on addressing the underlying etiology through appropriate dental treatment, with the aim of eliminating the source of pain. When analgesic administration is required, intramuscular administration should be avoided. Paracetamol (acetaminophen) is considered the analgesic of choice. The use of nonsteroidal anti-inflammatory drugs (NSAIDs) is not recommended, except for selective cyclooxygenase-2 (COX-2) inhibitors. For the management of more intense pain, oral opioids (tramadol, codeine, hydrocodone, etc.) may be used alone or in combination with paracetamol [2].

13.2 Oral Surgery in Persons with Hemophilia

Invasive dental procedures should be meticulously planned and require close cooperation between a hematologist and a dental specialist, ensuring comprehensive interdisciplinary assessment and risk management. The decision to proceed with oral surgical treatment should be made by specialists in mutual agreement and should include an assessment of preoperative and postoperative factors, as well as the need for hospitalization. The type and extent of the dental procedure, along with the severity of the disease, are key factors that influence the decision regarding the need for factor replacement therapy. Although not widely accepted, efforts have been made to develop specific tools for assessing bleeding risk and dental treatment in persons with hemophilia [32].

Oral surgical procedures in persons with hemophilia are considered high-risk because of prolonged, extensive postoperative bleeding. Such procedures require careful planning. Oral surgery should be performed with minimal trauma and the use of local hemostatic agents (oxidized regenerated cellulose, fibrin glue, collagen, and gelatin-based products) (Fig. 13.1), along with local hemostatic measures such

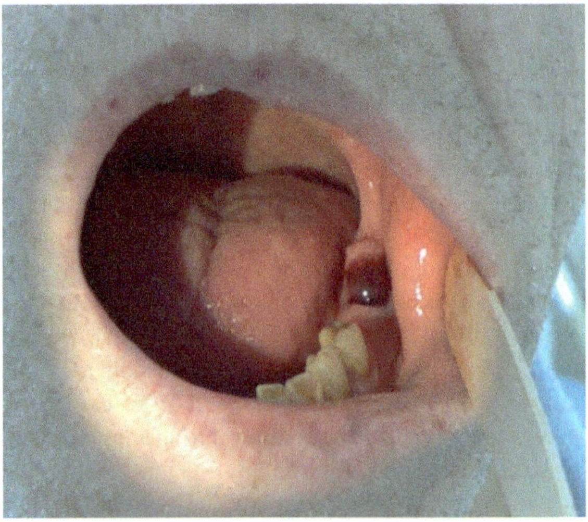

Fig. 13.1 Post-extraction wound in a person with haemophilia A and low-titer of inhibitors, 1 h after tooth extraction and fibrin glue application

as wound compression, suturing, and the use of a soft, vacuum-formed splint (see Chap. 27).

The therapeutic plan should also include a decision about whether the procedure will be performed in an outpatient (ambulatory surgery) or inpatient (hospital) setting. Nowadays, tooth extractions and other minor oral surgical procedures are commonly performed in an outpatient setting or as day-case procedures. Hospitalization is usually recommended for more extensive procedures, those performed under general anesthesia, procedures in persons with high-titer inhibitors, and those living far from a hospital without adequate support at home [1]. The procedure typically requires hematologic treatment, including the use of CFC and antifibrinolytic agents. In persons with mild hemophilia A who respond well, the use of DDAVP may be considered. Adherence to postoperative instructions is of great importance. Patients should be advised not to spit, suck, or rinse their mouths; to follow a soft, cold diet; to avoid smoking; and to brush their teeth gently for several days. Clear instructions regarding medications during the postoperative period are also necessary. Acetylsalicylic acid and other NSAIDs should be avoided. The use of acetaminophen or selective COX-2 inhibitors is recommended when postoperative analgesia is required. Antibiotic prophylaxis or therapy is reserved for strictly defined indications. Postoperatively, antifibrinolytics and antimicrobial mouth rinses, most commonly based on chlorhexidine gluconate, may be prescribed. Caution is required when using mouth rinses due to the risk of dislodging the blood clot. Bleeding in the head and neck region, particularly on the floor of the oral cavity, can be life-threatening. Therefore, patients should be instructed to report immediately to the hematologist or dentist on duty if they experience any prolonged bleeding, difficulty swallowing, or difficulty breathing. Patients should be given the phone number of a health caregiver to reach in case of postoperative bleeding [2].

Given that tooth extraction is by far the most common oral surgical procedure, it is understandable that the professional literature focuses most on achieving the safest possible approach to dental extraction in persons with hemophilia. However, despite the procedure's frequency, there is currently no consensus on the duration of hematological treatment or the optimal preoperative factor levels to prevent postoperative bleeding [1]. Various national and international guidelines [3, 4, 24, 25] provide general recommendations for the dental management of persons with hemophilia. However, there is no generally accepted hematological protocol for dentoalveolar surgical procedures.

A recently published review of the literature proposed hematological regimens for tooth extraction, classified into three groups: pre- and postoperative CFC or DDAVP, single preoperative CFC or DDAVP, and no factor replacement or DDAVP treatment [1]. The review included 11 studies in which persons with hemophilia A received CFC before and after tooth extraction, aiming to raise FVIII levels to 10%–50% or 50%–100%. In most of these studies, FVIII levels increased by >50% before tooth extraction, followed by the same or half a dose postoperatively for 1–3 days, in combination with systemic and/or local antifibrinolytic agents. In some of these studies, persons with mild hemophilia A were treated with DDAVP at a dose of 0.3 μg/kg. The overall reported postoperative bleeding rate was 11.9%, with a range of 3.9%–27.8%. In the 13 included studies, hematological treatment consisted solely of preoperative administration of CFC or DDAVP in cases of mild disease. In most of these studies, the aim was to raise FVIII to 30%–50% preoperatively. The overall reported bleeding rate for single use of CFC or DDAVP was 11.4% (range 2%–31.6%), which is similar to the frequency of postoperative bleeding in persons who received CFC preoperatively and postoperatively (11.4% vs 11.9%). The majority of authors recommend factor replacement therapy for tooth extraction. However, this review suggests that perioperative CFC use in persons with hemophilia can be reduced. A single preoperative dose of CFC is generally sufficient, and with the use of antifibrinolytics and local hemostatic measures, the risk of postoperative bleeding can be significantly minimized [1].

There are also several case reports and case series in which tooth extractions were performed without the use of factor replacement therapy, typically relying solely on antifibrinolytic treatment [28, 33, 34]. Because these studies involved small numbers of participants, typically those with a mild form of the disease [33], and in some of them patients on regular factor prophylaxis were included [28], it is not possible to draw firm conclusions regarding the justification and safety of this therapeutic approach [1]. The fact is that such a treatment protocol has not been sufficiently validated clinically, and additional caution is required, especially in cases where bleeding may be life-threatening, such as in the floor of the oral cavity.

The use of antifibrinolytic agents in oral surgical procedures is important, given the confirmed presence of plasminogen and its activators in saliva [35–37]. Delayed post-extraction bleeding is frequently observed in persons with hemophilia, typically occurring several days after tooth extraction, and is most commonly attributed to fibrinolysis of the blood clot (Fig. 13.2). The most commonly used antifibrinolytics are epsilon-aminocaproic acid (EACA) and tranexamic acid (TA). These drugs are plasminogen inhibitors and can be administered both systemically and locally. EACA is less commonly used than TA because of a shorter half-life, lower efficacy, and greater toxicity. TA is administered orally at a dose of 25 mg/kg, three to four times a day, with therapy typically lasting for 7 days. It can also be used intravenously at a dose of 10 mg/kg, two to three times a day [2, 4, 38]. Antifibrinolytic treatment should start before the planned oral surgery. These agents may also be used locally, either applied directly to the wound or as a mouthwash solution.

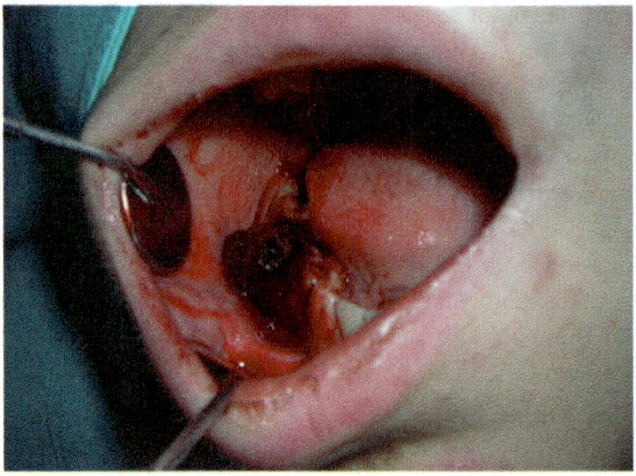

Fig. 13.2 Delayed post-extraction bleeding in a person with hemophilia A caused by fibrinolysis of the blood clot

Five percent TA is the most commonly used antifibrinolytic mouthwash solution, administered at a dose of 10 mL every 4–6 h for 5–7 days following the surgery [3, 4, 24, 25]. If used systemically, antifibrinolytics will show activity in the blood but not in saliva. If used locally, they will have an effect in saliva but not in the blood. Therefore, some authors advocate their use both locally and systemically [39]. The use of antifibrinolytic agents may reduce the need for factor replacement therapy or decrease the total dose of required CFC [2].

It should be noted that some people with hemophilia have blood-borne infections, such as HIV and hepatitis B and C. This is particularly common among those who were treated with blood products in the past. The mere presence of these infections does not affect dental treatment. However, in advanced or active stages of the disease, dental treatment must be adapted to the patient's overall medical condition. Universal precautions are essential to prevent the transmission of bloodborne diseases.

13.3 Oral Surgery in Persons with Hemophilia A and Hemophilia B with Inhibitors

Box 13.2 Dental Considerations in PwH and Inhibitors

1. *Low-responding inhibitor <5.0 BU*
2. *High-responding inhibitor ≥5.0 BU*

Oral surgery in PwH and inhibitors

- Thorough dental treatmant plan in discussion with a hematologist
- Bleeding control is a greater challenge in PwH and inhibitors than in those without inhibitors
- Inpatient treatment is recommended
- Inhibitor screening should be done preoperatively
- Perioperative hematological treatment depends on the risk of the procedure and level of antibodies and may include higher doses and more frequent FVIII or FIX concentrates, the use of bypassing agents (rFVIIa and aPCC) and antifibrinolytics
  - In PwH A and PwH B with low-responding inhibitors higher doses of FVIII or FIX products and more frequent dosing than usual are recommended
  - In PwH A and PwH B and high-responding inhibitors bypassing agents are recommended
  - In PwH B and high-responding FIX inhibitors with allergic reactions to FIX clotting factor concentrate rFVIIa is recommended instead of aPCC
  - Use of antifibrinolytics systemically and/or locally along with clotting factor concentrates or bypassing agents
  - Caution is necessary with concomitant antifibrinolytic and aPCC use
- For other recommendations see Box 13.1

BU- Bethesda units; F VIII- coagulation factor VIII; FIX-coagulation factor IX; PwH- person with hemophilia A or B; rFVIIa- activated recombinant FVII; aPCC- activated prothrombin complex concentrate

Dental management of persons with hemophilia and inhibitors may pose a significant clinical challenge. Given the high prevalence and preventability of oral diseases, it is of utmost importance to minimize the need for oral surgical procedures. Because of the increased risk of postoperative complications and the high cost of hematological treatment, oral surgical interventions in persons with inhibitors are typically performed in hospital settings. Hematological treatment usually involves the use of bypassing agents, such as activated prothrombin complex concentrate (aPCC) or activated recombinant FVII (rFVIIa). In persons with low-responding inhibitors (<5 BU/ml), high doses of CFC can be administered. However, in persons who respond inadequately to this therapy or have a high antibody titer ≥5 BU/ml (high-responders), this approach is not recommended. Instead, they are managed with bypassing agents. rFVIIa is typically administered as a bolus of 90–120 μg/kg immediately prior to the procedure, and due to its short half-life, repeated doses are given at 2–3 h after the intervention until adequate hemostasis is achieved. Antifibrinolytics are also important. aPCC is used in persons with hemophilia and inhibitors at a dose of 75–85 U/kg every 8–12 h, provided that the total daily dose does not exceed 200 U/kg [2, 40]. aPCC should not be used in persons with hemophilia B who have an allergic reaction to FIX, given that the product contains FIX and may provoke an allergic reaction. Caution is required when administering antifibrinolytics and aPCC due to the risk of thromboembolism [2]. Some persons with inhibitors respond better to rFVIIa, while others respond more favorably to aPCCs. Therefore, in cases of inadequate therapeutic response, it is necessary to consider changing the therapy. Combination of sequential bypass agent therapy is also a treatment option.

A recent review of the literature highlights the limited number of reported oral surgical procedures in persons with inhibitors [1]. The literature includes case series and case reports involving a small number of pediatric and adult patients with inhibitors who successfully underwent tooth extraction following hematologic treatment with rFVIIa or aPCC [41–45]. However, reports of severe bleeding can also be found, primarily involving hemorrhage into the floor of the mouth with potential airway obstruction, following tooth extraction in this group of patients [46, 47]. The lack of randomized studies with larger sample sizes, as well as the variability in hematological treatment protocols, prevent drawing firmer conclusions regarding the safest approach to oral surgical treatment in persons with hemophilia and inhibitors.

13.4 Oral Surgery in Persons with Hemophilia A Receiving Emicizumab Prophylaxis

Box 13.3 Dental Considerations in PwH A Receiving Emicizumab

1. *In PwH A and inhibitors regular prophylaxis with emicizumab is recommended*
2. *In persons with severe hemophilia A without inhibitors regular prophylaxis with emicizumab may be used*

Oral surgery in PwH A receiving emicizumab

- Thorough dental treatment plan in discussion with a hematologist
- Perioperative hematological treatment depends on the risk of the procedure and the presence of inhibitors and may include FVIII-containing product or bypassing agents and antifibrinolytics
  - In PwH A and inhibitors receiving emicizumab who undergo minor surgery either low-dose or no FVIII replacement is recommended
  - In PwH A and low-responding inhibitors receiving emicizumab who undergo major surgery FVIII concentrate is recommended
  - In PwH A and high-responding inhibitors receiving emicizumab who undergo major surgery rFVIIa is recommended. aPCC should be avoided due to the risk of thrombotic microangiopathy
  - Use of antifibrinolytics systemically and/or locally along with FVIII concentrate or rFVIIa
- For other recommendations see Box 13.1

PwH A person with hemophilia A, *rFVIIa* recombinant factor VIIa, *aPCC* activated prothrombin complex concentrate

The number of persons with hemophilia, both with and without inhibitors, receiving prophylaxis with emicizumab is increasing, and this trend is expected to continue. The introduction of emicizumab into clinical practice has raised new considerations regarding the perioperative management of these persons during elective surgical procedures. Emicizumab is effective in preventing bleeding but is not used to treat acute bleeding episodes. According to the World Federation of Hemophilia (WFH), in individuals receiving emicizumab prophylaxis, minor surgical procedures are generally recommended to be performed without factor replacement therapy or with low-dose CFC [2]. For extensive surgical procedures or those associated with a high risk of postoperative bleeding in persons receiving emicizumab prophylaxis, treatment depends on inhibitor titers. In persons with low-titer inhibitors (<5 BU/mL), frequent administration of high doses of CFC is recommended. For those with high-titer inhibitors (≥5 BU/mL), a bypassing agent is suggested, with a preference for rFVIIa over aPCC because of the risk of thrombotic microangiopathy [2].

Given that emicizumab has recently been introduced into clinical practice, there is limited data in the literature on perioperative management for oral surgery in these patients. The protocols that have typically been applied are usually based on the treating physician's discretion.

The HAVEN 1–4 studies [48] included persons with hemophilia A on emicizumab prophylaxis who required, among other procedures, 62 dental treatments, including 29 tooth extractions, 15 endodontic procedures, and 7 dental implant placements. Twenty-nine dental procedures were performed in persons with inhibitors, and 33 in those without inhibitors. Of the 62 procedures, 22 (35.5%) were performed with hemostatic cover, including 5 of 29 procedures in persons with inhibitors, for which rFVIIa was used, and 16 of 33 procedures in persons without inhibitors, for which standard- or extended-half-life CFC were administered. In most cases, single doses of rFVIIa (4 of 5) or FVIII CFC (13 of 16) were used. Forty dental procedures were performed without factor replacement therapy. Postoperative bleeding was recorded in 11 of 22 procedures with hemostatic cover. In five (22.7%) of these cases, bleeding was controlled with further hematological treatment. In persons without factor replacement therapy, postoperative bleeding occurred in 13 of 40 procedures, of which 9 (22.5%) required hematological treatment for bleeding control. Seventeen of 62 procedures were performed using only antifibrinolytic therapy, with no postoperative bleeding observed in 10 (58.8%) of these cases. The results of the study showed that both minor and major surgical procedures can be safely performed in persons with hemophilia A receiving emicizumab prophylaxis, with the use of FVIII CFC in persons without inhibitors or rFVIIa in those with inhibitors. For minor dental procedures, the use of factor replacement therapy was often not necessary. However, the importance of using antifibrinolytic therapy was also emphasized [48].

A similar conclusion was drawn from a review of the literature [49], which indicated that, depending on the extent of the oral surgical procedure, the treatment protocol for persons with hemophilia and inhibitors receiving emicizumab prophylaxis may include the use of bypassing agents in combination with antifibrinolytics or the sole use of antifibrinolytics. The level of inhibitor titers also plays a significant role in determining the hematological protocol [49].

A recent study [50] involved 10 persons receiving emicizumab prophylaxis who underwent 17 dental procedures, including 29 tooth extractions. Hemostatic cover varied by procedure, with some receiving only preoperative hemostatic cover, others receiving both pre- and postoperative hemostatic cover, and others receiving no factor replacement at all, depending on the extent of the procedure and the results of rotational thromboelastometry. In 8 persons with hemophilia A without inhibitors, 13 dental extraction procedures were performed, of which 10 received FVIII CFC, while 3 did not. In two persons with hemophilia A and inhibitors, a total of four dental extraction procedures were performed with the use of rFVIIa as hemostatic cover. The authors reported no cases of postoperative bleeding. The authors concluded that with appropriate systemic hematological treatment, assessment of coagulation status and procedural bleeding risk, and the proper use of local hemostatic agents and measures, oral surgery can be safely performed in persons with hemophilia, both with and without inhibitors, receiving emicizumab prophylaxis [50].

13.5 Dental Implant Placement in Persons with Hemophilia

The trauma associated with dental implant placement is comparable to that following tooth extraction. However, implant placement often requires additional procedures such as bone grafting, sinus lift, and soft tissue augmentation. When performing these procedures in people with bleeding disorders, a comprehensive treatment plan is required. Additional caution is also necessary during mandibular implant placement to avoid perforation of the lingual cortex, which may lead to hemorrhage with potentially life-threatening consequences in persons with hemophilia.

Implant placement in persons with hemophilia should be carried out with careful planning and analysis of cone beam computed tomography (CBCT) scans, with minimal trauma and the fewest number of surgical procedures. Certain implant placement and loading protocols could have significant advantages in patients with bleeding disorders. Immediate implant placement, i.e., the placement of implants at the time of tooth extraction, when indicated, may reduce the number of surgical procedures. A one-stage (non-submerged) surgical implant placement protocol avoids an additional surgical intervention and further manipulation of soft tissues. Immediate loading is feasible provided that primary implant stability is achieved. It is necessary to consider reducing trauma to the soft tissues and bone during implant placement. Soft tissue trauma may be minimized by avoiding flap reflection, i.e., by a "flapless" technique. Insufficient bone volume requires the use of bone augmentation procedures. These procedures are associated with higher morbidity and a prolonged healing period and therefore should not be considered as treatment options that should be given priority in persons with hemophilia [25]. If properly indicated, the use of short or extra short implants may serve as an alternative to more extensive bone grafting and sinus lift techniques [51].

There is limited data in the literature on implant placement in persons with hemophilia and other congenital coagulopathies [52]. Reports of single or a few cases of successful implant placement in persons with hemophilia A and hemophilia B are available [53–57]. In addition to the use of antifibrinolytics, proposed hematological protocols range from single preoperative factor replacement therapy, aimed at raising factor levels to approximately 40% [53, 54], to more intensive regimens involving both preoperative and postoperative factor administration, with the goal of raising FVIII levels to 100% preoperatively and 50% postoperatively [56] or maintaining levels between 80% and 100% both preoperatively and postoperatively for several days [57]. Gatti et al. [58] conducted a prospective study that included 10 persons with hemophilia, 8 with hemophilia A and 2 with hemophilia B, who had 21 implants placed during 15 surgical procedures. The hematological treatment involved CFC administration to raise factor levels above 50% preoperatively and to maintain factor levels above 30% postoperatively for up to 72 h following the procedure, with concurrent use of antifibrinolytics. Postoperative bleeding occurred in 3 of 15 cases, and all were easily controlled by local hemostatic measures. The authors reported that all implants were successfully osseointegrated after 4 months of follow-up [57].

Regarding bone augmentation procedures in the context of implant therapy in persons with hemophilia, the literature contains a limited number of case reports. Several case reports describe bone augmentation procedures using xenografts [53, 54], whereas case reports of bone autografts in persons with hemophilia are lacking. A case report of postoperative bleeding following a sinus lift and several implant placements in a person with mild hemophilia has been reported [59].

Despite the currently limited data in the literature, it can be reasonably assumed that dental implant procedures in patients with inherited bleeding disorders will be a focus in the future.

References

1. Bajkin B, Dougall A. Current state of play regarding dental extractions in patients with haemophilia: consensus or evidence-based practice? A review of the literature. Haemophilia. 2020;26(2):183–99.
2. Srivastava A, Santagostino E, Dougall A, Kitchen S, Sutherland M, Pipe SW, Carcao M, Mahlangu J, Ragni MV, Windyga J, Llinás A, Goddard NJ, Mohan R, Poonnoose PM, Feldman BM, Lewis SZ, van den Berg HM, Pierce GF, WFH Guidelines for the Management of Hemophilia Panelists, et al. WFH guidelines for the management of hemophilia, 3rd edition. Haemophilia. 2020;26(Suppl 6):1–158. Erratum in: Haemophilia 2021;27(4):699.
3. Brewer A, Correa ME. Guidelines for dental treatment of patients with inherited bleeding disorders. World Federation of Hemophilia Treatment of Hemophilia Monograph; 2006. Available from: http://www1.wfh.org/publications/files/pdf-1190.pdf. Accessed 2 Feb 2023.
4. Scully C, Diz Dios P, Giangrande P. Oral care for people with hemophilia or a hereditary bleeding tendency. World Federation of Hemophilia Treatment of Hemophilia Monograph; 2008. Available from: http://www1.wfh.org/publications/files/pdf-1164.pdf. Accessed 8 Feb 2023.
5. Mulders G, van Verseveld H, van der Geer J, Wolvius E, Leebeek F. The state of oral health in patients with haemophilia in the Netherlands. Haemophilia. 2023;29(2):466–78.
6. Kabil N, El Alfy M, Metwalli N. Evaluation of the oral health situation of a group of Egyptian haemophilic children and their re-evaluation following an oral hygiene and diet education programme. Haemophilia. 2007;13:287–92.
7. Azhar S, Yazdanie N, Muhammad N. Periodontal status and IOTN interventions among young hemophiliacs. Haemophilia. 2006;12:401–4.
8. Yazicioglu I, Deveci C, Çiftçi V, Antmen B, Doğan MC. Parent's report on oral health-related quality of life of children with haemophilia. Haemophilia. 2019;25(2):229–35.
9. Baskirt EA, Albayrak H, Ak G, Pinar Erdem A, Sepet E, Zulfikar B. Dental and periodontal health in children with haemophilia. J Coagul Disord. 2009;1:7–10.
10. Babu NV, Shah M, Patel P. Oral health status in children with haemophilia—a comparative study. J Haemophilia Prac. 2016;3:1–5.
11. Czajkowska S, Rupa-Matysek J, Gil L, Surdacka A. Assessment of oral health and healthy habits in adult patients with congenital hemophilia. Eur J Dent. 2023;17(1):161–72.
12. Rajantie H, Alapulli H, Mäkipernaa A, Ranta S. Oral health care in children with haemophilia in Helsinki, Finland. Eur Arch Paediatr Dent. 2013;14(5):339–43.
13. Kumar M, Pai KM, Kurien A, Vineetha R. Oral hygiene and dentition status in children and adults with hemophilia: a case-control study. Spec Care Dentist. 2018;38(6):391–4.
14. Mielnik-Blaszczak M. Evaluation of dentition status and oral hygiene in Polish children and adolescents with congenital hemorrhagic diatheses. Int J Paediatr Dent. 1999;9:99–103.
15. Othman NA, Sockalingam SN, Mahyuddin A. Oral health status in children and adolescents with haemophilia. Haemophilia. 2015;21(5):605–11.

16. Kanjani V, Annigeri RG, Hanagavadi S, Manjunath MR. Comparative analysis of oral health and treatment necessities in hemophilia individuals of Davangere population—a case control study. J Family Med Prim Care. 2020;9(9):4774–7.
17. Ziebolz D, Stühmer C, Hornecker E, Zapf A, Mausberg RF, Chenot JF. Oral health in adult patients with congenital coagulation disorders—a case control study. Haemophilia. 2011;17(3):527–31.
18. Sonbol H, Pelargidou M, Lucas VS, Gelbier MJ, Mason C, Roberts GJ. Dental health indices and caries-related microflora in children with severe haemophilia. Haemophilia. 2001;7(5):468–74.
19. Boyd D, Kinirons M. Dental caries experience of children with haemophilia in Northern Ireland. Int J Paediatr Dent. 1997;7:149–53.
20. Jangra B, Goswami M. Assessment of dental caries experience and periodontal health status among children with haemophilia in New Delhi, India—a case control study. Oral Health Prev Dent. 2017;15:131–7.
21. Salem K, Eshghi P. Dental health and oral health-related quality of life in children with congenital bleeding disorders. Haemophilia. 2013;19(1):65–70.
22. Žaliūnienė R, Aleksejūnienė J, Brukienė V, Pečiulienė V. Do hemophiliacs have a higher risk for dental caries than the general population? Medicina (Kaunas). 2015;51(1):46–56.
23. Brown MC, Hastie E, Shumake C, Waters B, Sidonio RF Jr. Dental habits and oral health in children and adolescents with bleeding disorders: a single-institution cross-sectional study. Haemophilia. 2022;28(1):73–9.
24. Anderson JA, Brewer A, Creagh D, Hook S, Mainwaring J, McKernan A, Yee TT, Yeung CA. Guidance on the dental management of patients with haemophilia and congenital bleeding disorders. Br Dent J. 2013;215:497–504.
25. Hewson ID, Daly J, Hallett KB, Liberali SA, Scott CL, Spaile G, Widmer R, Winters J. Consensus statement by hospital based dentists providing dental treatment for patients with inherited bleeding disorders. Aust Dent J. 2011;56(2):221–6.
26. Little JW, Miller CS, Rhodus NL. Congenital bleeding and hypercoagulable disorders. In: Little and Falace's sdental management of the medically compromised patient. 9th ed. St. Louis: Elsevier; 2018. p. 457–79.
27. Nanayakkara L, Yahaya N, Parreira M, Bajkin B. Dental management of people with complex or rare inherited bleeding disorders. Haemophilia. 2024;30(Suppl 3):128–34.
28. Hewson I, Makhmalbaf P, Street A, McCarthy P, Walsh M. Dental surgery with minimal factor support in the inherited bleeding disorder population at the Alfred Hospital. Haemophilia. 2011;17(1):e185–8.
29. Bartlett G, Mansoor J. Articaine buccal infiltration vs lidocaine inferior dental block—a review of the literature. Br Dent J. 2016;220(3):117–20.
30. Almadhoon HW, Abuiriban RW, Almassri H, Al-Hamed FS. Efficacy of 4% articaine buccal infiltration versus inferior alveolar nerve block for mandibular molars with symptomatic Irreversible pulpitis: A systematic review and meta-analysis. J Evid Based Dent Pract. 2022;22(2):101712.
31. Dougall A, Apperley O, Smith G, Madden L, Parkinson L, Daly B. Safety of buccal infiltration local anaesthesia for dental procedures. Haemophilia. 2019;25(2):270–5.
32. Rasaratnam L, Chowdary P, Pollard D, Subel B, Harrington C, Darbar UR. Risk-based management of dental procedures in patients with inherited bleeding disorders: development of a dental bleeding risk assessment and treatment tool (DeBRATT). Haemophilia. 2017;23(2):247–54.
33. Lewandowski B, Wojnar J, Brodowski R, Mucha M, Czenczek-Lewandowska E, Brzecka D. Dental extractions in patients with mild hemophilia A and hemophilia B and von Willebrand disease without clotting factor supplementation. Pol Arch Intern Med. 2018;128:7–8.
34. Bajkin BV, Rajic NV, Vujkov SB. Dental extraction in a hemophilia patient without factor replacement therapy: a case report. J Oral Maxillofac Surg. 2012;70:2276–7.
35. Sindet-Pedersen S, Gram J, Jespersen J. Characterization of plasminogen activators in unstimulated and stimulated human whole saliva. J Dent Res. 1987;66:1199–203.

36. Gersel-Pedersen N. Fibrinolytic activity of blood and saliva before and after oral surgery. Int J Oral Surg. 1981;10(Suppl 1):114–21.
37. Majerus P, Dalcette B, Hermans M, Pourtois M, Capel P. Variations in fibrinolytic activity of human whole saliva. Eur J Oral Sci. 1996;104:341–5.
38. Arruda VR, High KA. Coagulation disorders. In: Harrison's principles of internal medicine. 20th ed. McGraw-Hill Education eBook; 2018. p. 830–8.
39. Sindet-Pedersen S, Stenbjerg S. Effect of local antifibrinolytic treatment with tranexamic acid in hemophiliacs undergoing oral surgery. J Oral Maxillofac Surg. 1986;44:703–7.
40. Brewer A. Dental management of patients with inhibitors to factor VIII or factor IX. World Federation of Hemophilia Treatment of Hemophilia Monograph; 2008. Available from: http://www1.wfh.org/publications/files/pdf-1200.pdf. Accessed 14 Feb 2023.
41. Laguna P, Klukowska A. Management of oral bleedings with recombinant factor VIIa in children with haemophilia A and inhibitor. Haemophilia. 2005;11(1):2–4.
42. Lauroua P, Ferrer AM, Guérin V. Successful major and minor surgery using factor VIII inhibitor bypassing activity in patients with haemophilia A and inhibitors. Haemophilia. 2009;15(6):1300–7.
43. Morimoto Y, Yoshioka A, Shima M, Kirita T. Intraoral hemostasis using a recombinant activated factor VII preparation in a hemophilia a patient with inhibitor. J Oral Maxillofac Surg. 2003;61(9):1095–7.
44. Windyga J, Stefanska-Windyga E, Odnoczko E, Baran B, Czubak G. Activated prothrombin complex concentrate in combination with tranexamic acid: a single centre experience for the treatment of mucosal bleeding and dental extraction in haemophilia patients with inhibitors. Haemophilia. 2016;22(5):e465–8.
45. Zanon E, Brandolin B, Saggiorato G, Bacci C. Complex dental extractions in a patient with severe haemophilia A and inhibitors treated with activated prothrombin complex concentrate. Blood Transfus. 2012;10(2):225–7.
46. Heiland M, Weber M, Schmelzle R. Life-threatening bleeding after dental extraction in a hemophilia A patient with inhibitors to factor VIII: a case report. J Oral Maxillofac Surg. 2003;61(11):1350–3.
47. Brkovic B, Jurisic M, Suvajdzic N, Rakic M, Mikovic D. Extensive bleeding after tooth extraction in patient with inhibitors to factor VIII: a case report. Haemophilia. 2010;16(Suppl. 4):11FP07.
48. Kruse-Jarres R, Peyvandi F, Oldenburg J, Chang T, Chebon S, Doral MY, Croteau SE, Lambert T, Kempton CL, Pipe SW, Ko RH, Trzaskoma B, Dhalluin C, Bienz NS, Niggli M, Lehle M, Paz-Priel I, Young G, Jiménez-Yuste V. Surgical outcomes in people with hemophilia A taking emicizumab prophylaxis: experience from the HAVEN 1–4 studies. Blood Adv. 2022;6(24):6140–50.
49. Jiménez-Yuste V, Rodríguez-Merchán EC, Matsushita T, Holme PA. Concomitant use of bypassing agents with emicizumab for people with haemophilia A and inhibitors undergoing surgery. Haemophilia. 2021;27(4):519–30.
50. Yagyuu T, Furukawa S, Zaizen M, Yata S, Imada M, Nogami K, Kirita T. Peri-operative hemostatic management of tooth extraction in patients with hemophilia A, with and without inhibitors, receiving emicizumab prophylaxis. Haemophilia. 2023;29(1):172–9.
51. Bajkin B. The potential significance of minimally invasive oral surgery and dental implant placement techniques in persons with inherited bleeding disorders. Haemophilia. 2022;28:56.
52. Römer P, Heimes D, Pabst A, Becker P, Thiem DGE, Kämmerer PW. Bleeding disorders in implant dentistry: a narrative review and a treatment guide. Int J Implant Dent. 2022;8(1):20.
53. Bacci C, Cerrato A, Zanette G, Pasca S, Zanon E. Regenerative surgery with dental implant rehabilitation in a haemophiliac patient. TH Open. 2021;5(1):e104–6.
54. Calvo-Guirado JL, Romanos GE, Delgado-Ruiz RA. Infected tooth extraction, bone grafting, immediate implant placement and immediate temporary crown insertion in a patient with severe type-B hemophilia. BMJ Case Rep. 2019;12(3):e229204.

55. Neskoromna Jędrzejczak A, Bogusiak K, Chojnowski K, Robak M, Treliński J. Implanto prosthetic rehabilitation of a patient with severe form of hemophilia B: a case report. Acta Haematol Pol. 2018;49(1):33–6.
56. Gornitsky M, Hammouda W, Rosen H. Rehabilitation of a hemophiliac with implants: a medical perspective and case report. J Oral Maxillofac Surg. 2005;63(5):592–7.
57. Castellanos-Cosano L, Núñez-Vázquez RJ, Segura-Egea JJ, Torres-Lagares D, Corcuera-Flores JR, Machuca-Portillo G. Protocol for oral implant rehabilitation in a hemophilic HIV-positive patient with type C hepatitis. Implant Dent. 2014;23(5):622–5.
58. Gatti PC, Parreira M, Gutierrez Fillol A, Gualtieri A, Puia SA. Prospective observational study on the clinical behaviour of dental implants in patients with haemophilia. Preliminary results. Br J Oral Maxillofac Surg. 2022;60(2):157–61.
59. de Azevedo KM, Brondani LP, de Mattos Carpena ALM, Dos Santos MBF. Delayed bleeding in a hemophilic patient after sinus floor elevation and multiple implant placements: a case report. J Oral Implantol. 2022;48(2):133–8.

Bleeding Disorders and Liver Disease

14

Branislav V. Bajkin and Ivana Urosevic

Liver diseases are diverse in etiology, with the most common causes including viral hepatitis B and C, chronic excessive alcohol consumption, autoimmune mechanisms, and steatohepatitis. In some cases, the underlying cause of impaired liver function cannot be identified. Hepatocellular damage can be acute, in which case liver function usually recovers after the underlying cause is eliminated and appropriate treatment is initiated. Chronic liver disease leads to irreversible impairment of liver function, replacement of hepatocytes with fibrous tissue, and the development of cirrhosis. Decompensated cirrhosis is accompanied by further complications and clinically presents with jaundice, portal hypertension, ascites, splenomegaly, esophageal varices, and hepatic encephalopathy.

The liver performs multiple functions within the hemostatic system. It synthesizes numerous procoagulant factors and anticoagulant proteins (antithrombin, proteins C and S) and components of the fibrinolytic system [1]. The liver synthesizes vitamin K-dependent coagulation factors (FII, FVII, FIX, FX), as well as certain coagulation factors that do not require vitamin K (FV, FXI, FXII, FXIII, and fibrinogen). Additionally, it synthesizes thrombopoietin, which regulates platelet production from megakaryocytes. In compensated liver disease, there is a decrease in both procoagulant and anticoagulant factors, typically resulting in a "rebalanced hemostasis" [2, 3]. This term refers to the functionality of the hemostatic system within a narrow scope. Such a state is extremely sensitive, and even minimal stress can disrupt its balance.

Liver dysfunction leads to complex impairment of the hemostatic system and a bleeding tendency due to decreased synthesis of coagulation factors, accelerated

B. V. Bajkin (✉)
University of Novi Sad, Faculty of Medicine, Dentistry Clinic of Vojvodina, Novi Sad, Serbia
e-mail: branislav.bajkin@mf.uns.ac.rs

I. Urosevic
University of Novi Sad, Faculty of Medicine, University Clinical Center of Vojvodina, Clinic of Hematology, Novi Sad, Serbia

B. V. Bajkin (ed.), *Bleeding Disorders and Dentistry*,
https://doi.org/10.1007/978-3-032-26713-9_14

fibrinolysis, and thrombocytopenia. Thrombocytopenia in patients with liver disease is usually moderate (50–100 × 10^9/L) and is caused by congestive splenomegaly and accelerated platelet sequestration, a shortened platelet lifespan (due to autoimmune destruction or decreased platelet production) because of impaired thrombopoietin synthesis or alcohol-induced bone marrow suppression [1–3]. Bleeding may be further exacerbated by dysfibrinogenemia and the development of disseminated intravascular coagulation (DIC).

In patients with liver disease, preoperative hemostasis assessment is essential. Laboratory test results depend on the severity of liver disease and typically show prolonged prothrombin time (PT), activated partial thromboplastin time (aPTT), and thrombin time (TT), thrombocytopenia, dysfibrinogenemia, and normal or slightly elevated levels of fibrin degradation products [1, 4]. Given the complexity of impairment of the hemostatic system in patients with liver disease, as well as impaired synthesis of both procoagulant and anticoagulant factors, it is important to emphasize that no single laboratory test reliably predicts the risk of postoperative bleeding.

In patients with advanced liver disease, thrombosis can also occur. Thrombosis most commonly affects the portal and mesenteric veins due to reduced portal blood flow and a hypercoagulable state. In these patients, laboratory findings often show elevated levels of von Willebrand factor (VWF) and FVIII, along with decreased levels of plasminogen and anticoagulant proteins, such as protein C, protein S, and antithrombin [1].

Child-Pugh and Model for End-Stage Liver Disease (MELD) scores are used to assess the severity of liver insufficiency. The Child-Pugh score indicates the degree of disease progression and includes the following parameters: ascites, encephalopathy, bilirubin and albumin levels, and INR (PT). Each parameter is individually scored one, two, or three points, and patients are classified into one of three classes: class A, mild liver disease (score 5–6); class B, moderate liver disease (score 7–9); and class C, end-stage liver disease (score 10–15). Higher scores indicate more severe disease [3]. The MELD score is used to assess priority for liver transplantation and includes the following parameters: serum levels of creatinine, bilirubin, sodium, and INR (PT) [3, 5]. Neither of these two scores is used to assess the need for transfusion preoperatively.

In patients with liver disease, fresh frozen plasma (FFP) is usually administered for bleeding. FFP at a dose of 5–10 mL/kg increases coagulation factor levels by approximately 10–20% [1]. The main side effect of FFP administration is volume overload. Prothrombin complex concentrate may be used as an alternative to FFP, though caution is advised because of the potential risk of thromboembolic complications [6]. Platelet concentrate is administered in cases of bleeding when the platelet count is typically below 10–20 × 10^9/L, preoperatively when the platelet count is below 50 × 10^9/L [1], or below 30–40 × 10^9/L for minor oral surgical procedures [5] (see Chap. 8). Preoperative prophylactic administration of FFP to correct prolonged PT should be done with caution, as it may disrupt the delicate "rebalanced hemostasis" that may exist in patients with compensated liver disease. Other treatment options include cryoprecipitate and fibrinogen concentrate, activated recombinant

FVII (rFVIIa), antifibrinolytics, and thrombopoietin receptor agonists [7]. The administration of vitamin K has limited or no effect because impaired liver function prevents its effective use.

References

1. Arruda VR, High KA. Coagulation disorders. In: Harrison's principles of internal medicine. 20th ed. McGraw-Hill Education eBook; 2018. p. 830–8.
2. Bermudez P, Beushausen M, Horan MP. Management of inherited, acquired, and iatrogenically induced coagulopathies in oral surgery. In: A textbook of advanced oral and maxillofacial surgery, vol. 3. InTech; 2016. p. 175–210.
3. Ephros H, Garibyan IL. Review of liver disease and perioperative management in dentistry. In: Szumita RP, Szumita PM, editors. Hemostasis in dentistry. Springer eBook; 2018. p. 52–60.
4. Scully C. Haemathology. In: Scully's medical problems in dentistry. 7th ed. Elsevier: Churchill Livingstone; 2014. p. 212–75.
5. Khanna S. Liver diseases. In: Meara DJ, Gutta R, editors. Oral and maxillofacial surgery for the medically compromised patients. Springer; 2022. p. 23–31.
6. Evans CR, Cuker A, Crowther M, Pishko AM. Prophylactic fresh frozen plasma versus prothrombin complex concentrate for preprocedural management of the coagulopathy of liver disease: a systematic review. Res Pract Thromb Haemost. 2022;6(4):e12724.
7. Roberts LN, Lisman T, Stanworth S, Hernandez-Gea V, Magnusson M, Tripodi A, Thachil J. Periprocedural management of abnormal coagulation parameters and thrombocytopenia in patients with cirrhosis: Guidance from the SSC of the ISTH. J Thromb Haemost. 2022;20(1):39–47.

Dental Management of Patients with Liver Disease

15

Branislav V. Bajkin and Alison Dougall

Box 15.1 Dental Management of Patients with Hepatic Insufficiency
General considerations

- Take universal precautions in patients with hepatitis B or hepatitis C infections
- Avoid the drugs that require liver metabolism
- Limit the total amount of local anesthetic solution
- Eliminate all dental foci in pretransplant liver patient

Oral surgery in patients with hepatic insufficiency

- Consult the patient's physician
- Inpatient or outpatient treatment depending on the bleeding risk of the procedure
- Preoperative laboratory screening (platelet count, prothrombin time, activated partial thromboplastin time, and bleeding time)
- Consider preoperative hematological treatment with fresh-frozen plasma or platelet transfusion depending on the extensiveness of surgery and laboratory findings (INR >3; platelet count <30.000)[a]
- Avoid situations in which the patient might swallow large amounts of blood
- Schedule a patient at the beginning of the work week
- Use of local anesthesia with vasoconstrictor

(continued)

B. V. Bajkin (✉)
University of Novi Sad, Faculty of Medicine, Dentistry Clinic of Vojvodina, Novi Sad, Serbia
e-mail: branislav.bajkin@mf.uns.ac.rs

A. Dougall
School of Dental Science, Trinity College Dublin, Dublin Dental University Hospital, Dublin, Ireland

B. V. Bajkin (ed.), *Bleeding Disorders and Dentistry*,
https://doi.org/10.1007/978-3-032-26713-9_15

Box 15.1 (continued)

- Minimally traumatic surgical technique; in case of multiple tooth extractions, consider quadrant oral surgery to minimize trauma
- Use of local hemostatic agents and measures to control oral bleeding
- For pain relief, use acetaminophen for short period of time (<2 weeks); avoid aspirin and other NSAIDs
- Provide a patient with postoperative instructions (soft and cold diet, phone number in case of an emergency) and regular follow-up

INR International Normalized Ratio, *NSAIDs* nonsteroidal anti-inflammatory drugs

[a]There is no general consensus regarding preoperative hematological treatment, and in many cases, it is not necessary. If used, the treatment goal is not to normalize hemostatic parameters prior to the procedure

Dental procedures in patients with liver disease may pose significant clinical challenges. The liver performs numerous vital functions in the body, many of which can affect dental treatment. The liver is responsible for metabolizing numerous drugs, including amide local anesthetics, certain antibiotics, and analgesics, which are the medications most commonly used in dentistry. This metabolism is of particular importance. Liver dysfunction also affects the hemostatic system, leading to an increased tendency for bleeding during invasive dental procedures. Additionally, delayed wound healing after oral surgical procedures and a reduced capacity to metabolize ingested blood should be considered in these patients.

For any invasive dental procedure in these patients, it is essential to obtain a detailed medical history, conduct a clinical examination, perform laboratory testing, and consult the patient's physician. It is particularly important to determine the underlying cause of liver dysfunction, especially given the relevance of blood-borne infections such as hepatitis B and hepatitis C in dental practice. Intraoral examination may reveal petechiae, gingival bleeding, and icteric and erythematous changes in the mucosa (Fig. 15.1a, b).

Previous bleeding episodes and laboratory tests may indicate the risk of operative bleeding (Fig. 15.2). However, accurate assessment of postoperative bleeding risk based solely on laboratory parameters is challenging, given the complex impairment of the hemostatic system in liver diseases. The most commonly used tests to assess hemostatic function in patients with liver disease are platelet count, prothrombin time (PT), and activated partial thromboplastin time (aPTT). INR (PT) is considered a good predictor of bleeding risk in patients taking oral anticoagulant therapy; however, in patients with liver disease, even slightly elevated INR values can be associated with a high risk of bleeding, given other factors that contribute to such risk. Thrombocytopenia also needs to be considered within the broader context of hemostatic dysfunction. There are some recent assays for the evaluation of

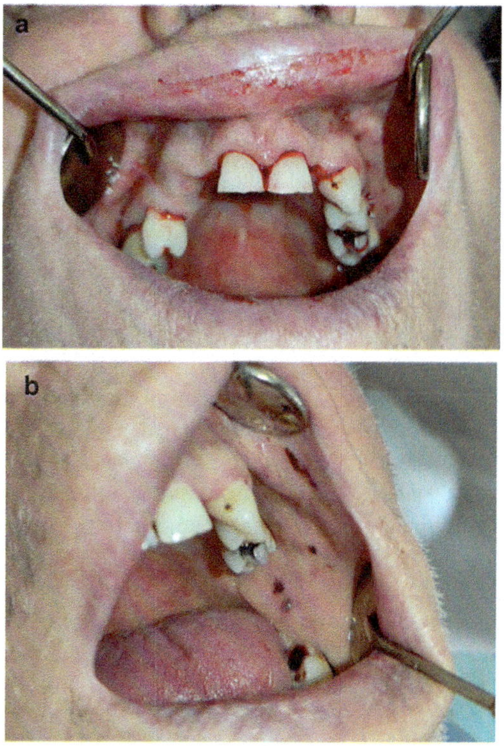

Fig. 15.1 (**a**, **b**) Gingival and oral mucosal bleeding in a patient with liver cirrhosis

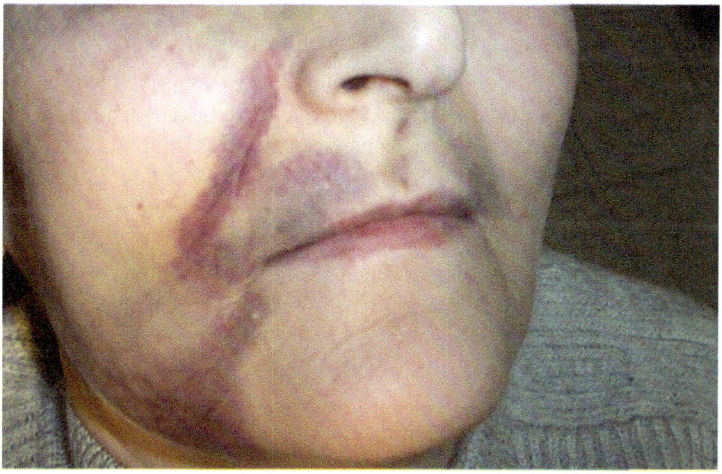

Fig. 15.2 Facial hematoma following tooth extraction in a patient with liver cirrhosis

hemostatic function, such as thromboelastography, thromboelastometry, and the thrombin generation test; however, their predictive value in assessing bleeding risk is still being examined [1, 2].

Consultation with the patient's physician improves the accuracy of the assessment of postoperative bleeding risk and facilitates the development of the optimal and safest treatment plan for these patients.

Based on the severity of the disease, laboratory findings, and the extent of the oral surgical procedure, a decision must be made regarding the preoperative use of systemic hemostatic agents, such as fresh-frozen plasma (FFP) or platelet concentrates, and whether the procedure should be performed in an outpatient or inpatient setting. It should be emphasized that complete preoperative normalization of hemostatic laboratory parameters is not the goal of systemic therapy and is often unnecessary. Surgical trauma should be minimized to reduce the risk of bleeding. When multiple teeth are extracted, the procedure can be limited to one quadrant per appointment [3]. Local hemostatic measures and agents are also important (see Chap. 27).

Results of several studies indicate that the risk of bleeding after tooth extraction is minimal at INR values <2.5 and platelet counts >30 × 10^9/L [4] or >40 × 10^9/L [5], without the preoperative use of FFP or platelet concentrate. Cocero et al. [5], in a retrospective study of 318 patients with liver disease who required 1183 tooth extractions, reported postoperative bleeding in 10 out of 318 patients (3.1%) or in 12 out of 1183 extracted teeth (1%). In the group of patients with defined INR values <2.5 and platelet counts >40 × 10^9/L, bleeding was observed in 1 of 271 patients (0.4%), which is comparable to the bleeding frequency reported in the general population. The remaining cases of bleeding were recorded in 9 out of 47 patients in total, of which 6 out of 44 patients had either INR values or platelet counts above the defined range, and finally, 3 out of 3 patients had INR values above 2.5 and platelet counts below 40 × 10^9/L [5].

Franco et al. [2] concluded that, compared with healthy individuals, patients with liver cirrhosis had greater blood loss following tooth extraction; however, the procedure can be considered safe even without preoperative prophylactic use of blood or blood products. The study included 74 participants in each group. The results also showed that standard laboratory tests, such as platelet count, INR (PT), aPTT, thrombin time (TT), platelet aggregation test, fibrinogen, protein C, protein S, antithrombin, and von Willebrand factor (VWF) level and activity, have little value in predicting postoperative bleeding risk [2]. Similar conclusions were reached by Medina et al. [6] in a retrospective study of patients with liver disease who underwent tooth extractions during 190 visits, without any hematologic treatment. Platelet counts ranged from 16 to 216 × 10^9/L, while reported INR values were <3. In 12 of 190 visits (6.31%), an equal frequency of intraoperative and postoperative bleeding was recorded. Intraoperative bleeding was more frequent in patients with a low platelet count, but laboratory tests did not prove reliable predictors of postoperative bleeding risk. All cases of bleeding were easily controlled by local hemostatic measures. The authors concluded that tooth extraction in patients with liver cirrhosis and a platelet count >16 × 10^9/L and INR values <3 is safe and does not require preoperative transfusion [6]. In contrast to studies reporting a low incidence of post-extraction bleeding in patients with liver disease who did not undergo preoperative hematologic treatment, the literature also describes cases of severe postoperative bleeding following tooth extraction that required the use of systemic hemostatic agents and treatment in a hospital setting [7].

In addition to studies conducted without preoperative hematological treatment, there are also those in which patients received transfusions prior to oral surgery. In most of these studies, the benefits of preoperative administration of FFP and/or platelet concentrates in cases of laboratory hemostatic abnormalities were not clearly confirmed. Postoperative bleeding was observed in both patients who received preoperative transfusions and those who did not [8–11]. These studies also indicated that routine laboratory tests, such as INR (PT), platelet count, and aPTT, are not good predictors of postoperative bleeding risk. As potential risk factors for postoperative bleeding, some authors identify degree of operative trauma [8], alcoholic liver cirrhosis and Child-Pugh class C [9], higher MELD score values [10], a positive medical history of previous postoperative bleeding, and a platelet count $<50 \times 10^9$/L [11].

A recently published systematic review of the literature on dental extraction in patients with liver cirrhosis included seven studies [12]. The total number of patients in these studies ranged from 23 to 318; the total number of extracted teeth ranged from 62 to 1183; platelet counts ranged from 16 to 216×10^9/L; and INR values were <4. The analysis of these studies showed that the incidence of post-extraction bleeding ranged from 0% to 8.9%, and almost all cases of bleeding were easily controlled by local hemostatic measures [12].

The number of published studies is insufficient, and the designs are heterogeneous, making it difficult to draw firm conclusions about a standardized protocol for oral surgical procedures in patients with liver disease. Standard laboratory hemostatic tests such as INR (PT), aPTTT, and platelet count are not considered relevant for predicting postoperative bleeding risk. However, in the absence of more reliable predictors, preoperative determination of these hemostatic parameters is recommended. There is no strong evidence that prophylactic preoperative administration of FFP and platelet concentrates can significantly prevent post-extraction bleeding [8–11]. Despite the small number of studies, the available research confirms that tooth extraction can be considered safe in patients without preoperative transfusions [2, 4–6]. However, a preoperative assessment of the patient's overall health condition is necessary. The prior experience of the entire team involved in the dental care of these patients is of great importance.

The use of aspirin and nonsteroidal anti-inflammatory drugs (NSAIDs) for managing postoperative pain should be avoided. These drugs are metabolized in the liver and have antithrombotic effects, which can cause erosions and ulcerations of the gastric mucosa. Acetaminophen is the analgesic of choice, but its use is recommended for a short period (<2 weeks) because of potential hepatotoxicity [3, 4, 13]. Because amide local anesthetics are metabolized in the liver, the total administered dose should be limited. In addition, because sedatives and anxiolytics are metabolized more slowly, caution and slow titration are necessary during dental procedures performed under general anesthesia [13].

The possibility of delayed wound healing and an increased risk of postoperative infection following tooth extraction should also be considered in patients with liver disease. Cocero et al. [14] investigated the need for antibiotic prophylaxis in patients who were candidates for liver transplantation. The study included 346 patients who underwent 662 oral surgical procedures, including 1329 extracted teeth. No cases of postoperative wound infection were recorded during the 7-day follow-up period, nor were any signs of systemic infection observed during the 14-day follow-up after the procedure. The authors concluded that antibiotic prophylaxis is not indicated for tooth extraction in patients with liver disease [14]. In patients at risk of developing spontaneous bacterial peritonitis, and in cases where a dental procedure is considered a potential contributing factor, consultation with the physician regarding antibiotic prophylaxis is recommended. Beta-lactam antibiotics are considered safe when antibiotic therapy for odontogenic infections is required, as they are eliminated via the kidneys [13].

15.1 Dental Management of Liver Transplant Patients

Patients who require liver transplantation or have already undergone the procedure are of particular interest. Liver transplantation is the only therapeutic option for end-stage liver disease. Because liver function is severely impaired, the risk of complications after dental procedures in these patients is significantly higher than in those with relatively preserved hepatic function. All dental foci must be diagnosed and eliminated before liver transplantation [3, 5, 9, 15]. Local infection in the oral cavity may contribute to the progression of liver disease through systemic inflammation. Some studies suggest a potential association between periodontal disease and liver disease, but further research is needed to confirm this [16, 17]. Immunosuppressive therapy administered in the posttransplantation period may exacerbate existing local infections, affecting postoperative morbidity and mortality.

During the immediate posttransplantation period, particularly within the first 3 months, only urgent dental procedures are indicated, and elective treatments should be postponed. Due to immunosuppressive therapy and the risk of organ rejection, antibiotic prophylaxis may be indicated for oral surgical procedures. Patients should be informed about the importance of oral hygiene and the potential development of gingival hyperplasia as a result of immunosuppressive therapy. Antibiotics should be used with caution in these patients because of the risk of developing fungal infections in the oral cavity. Also, caution is needed when prescribing drugs metabolized in the liver. In cases of acute or chronic graft rejection, dental interventions should be limited to urgent procedures only. If an oral surgical procedure cannot be postponed, assessment of hemostatic status and antibiotic prophylaxis are necessary [1, 13].

References

1. Ephros H, Garibyan IL. Review of liver disease and perioperative management in dentistry. In: Szumita RP, Szumita PM, editors. Hemostasis in dentistry. Springer eBook; 2018. p. 52–60.
2. Franco JB, Andrade NS, Bueno MVRDS, Peres MPSM, Medina JB, Tenório JDR, Rech BO, Ortega KL. Assessment of laboratory tests and intraoperative bleeding in patients with

liver cirrhosis undergoing tooth extractions. Oral Surg Oral Med Oral Pathol Oral Radiol. 2022;133(2):148–55.
3. Khanna S. Liver diseases. In: Meara DJ, Gutta R, editors. Oral and maxillofacial surgery for the medically compromised patients. Springer; 2022. p. 23–31.
4. Perdigão JPV. Postoperative bleeding after dental extraction in liver pretransplant patients. J Oral Maxillofac Surg. 2012;70:e177–84.
5. Cocero N, Bezzi M, Martini S, Carossa S. Oral surgical treatment of patients with chronic liver disease: assessments of bleeding and its relationship with thrombocytopenia and blood coagulation parameters. J Oral Maxillofac Surg. 2017;75(1):28–34.
6. Medina JB, Andrade NS, de Paula EF, Bezinelli L, Franco JB, Gallottini M, Braz-Silva PH, Ortega KL. Bleeding during and after dental extractions in patients with liver cirrhosis. Int J Oral Maxillofac Surg. 2018;47(12):1543–9.
7. Thomson PJ, Langton SG. Persistent haemorrhage following dental extractions in patients with liver disease: two cautionary tales. Br Dent J. 1996;180:141–4.
8. Ward BB, Weideman EM. Long-term postoperative bleeding after dentoalveolar surgery in the pretransplant liver failure patient. J Oral Maxillofac Surg. 2006;64:1469–74.
9. Niederhagen B, Wolff M, Appel T, von Lindern JJ, Bergé S. Location and sanitation of dental foci in liver transplantation. Transpl Int. 2003;16(3):173–8.
10. Helenius-Hietala J, Åberg F, Meurman JH, Nordin A, Isoniemi H. Oral surgery in liver transplant candidates: a retrospective study on delayed bleeding and other complications. Oral Surg Oral Med Oral Pathol Oral Radiol. 2016;121(5):490–5.
11. Souza AF, Rocha AL, Silva RKM, Bemquerer LM, Lanza CRM, Castro WH, Abreu LG, Silva TA, Travassos DV. Hemorrhagic complications in individuals with liver disease submitted to minor oral surgery. Blood Coagul Fibrinolysis. 2022;33(7):412–7.
12. de Oliveira RB, Rocha Tenório J, Bertoldi Franco J, Medina JB, Gallottini M, Pérez-Sayáns M, Ortega KL. Risk of bleeding during oral surgery in patients with liver cirrhosis: a systematic review. J Am Dent Assoc. 2021;152(1):46–54.e2.
13. Douglas LR, Douglass JB, Sieck JO, Smith PJ. Oral management of the patient with end-stage liver disease and the liver transplant patient. Oral Surg Oral Med Oral Pathol Oral Radiol Endod. 1998;86(1):55–64.
14. Cocero N, Frascolino C, Berta GN, Carossa S. Is it safe to remove teeth in liver transplant patients without antibiotics? A retrospective study of 346 patients. J Oral Maxillofac Surg. 2019;77(8):1557–65.
15. Glassman P, Wong C, Gish R. A review of liver transplantation for the dentist and guidelines for dental management. Spec Care Dentist. 1993;13(2):74–80.
16. Chen Y, Yang YC, Zhu BL, Wu CC, Lin RF, Zhang X. Association between periodontal disease, tooth loss and liver diseases risk. J Clin Periodontol. 2020;47(9):1053–63.
17. Wijarnpreecha K, Panjawatanan P, Cheungpasitporn W, Lukens FJ, Harnois DM, Pungpapong S, Ungprasert P. The association between periodontitis and nonalcoholic fatty liver disease: a systematic review and meta-analysis. J Gastrointestin Liver Dis. 2020;29(2):211–7.

Hemostasis and Malignant Diseases

16

Branislav V. Bajkin and Ivana Urosevic

The impact of malignant diseases on the hemostatic system is complex and may manifest as either a hypercoagulable state or an increased bleeding tendency. A hypercoagulable state is primarily associated with a predisposition to venous thrombosis but may also involve arterial thrombosis, often requiring antithrombotic therapy. Trousseau syndrome, also known as *thrombophlebitis migrans*, refers to recurrent thrombophlebitis at various sites and may be an early sign of malignancy. The underlying mechanism of hemostatic dysfunction in patients with malignant diseases is complex and primarily involves malignant cells (solid tumors), increased levels of tissue procoagulant factors and inflammatory cytokines, and other coagulation factors, fibrinogen, the fibrinolytic system, and platelets [1]. Additionally, the tendency toward thromboembolic complications can be influenced by immunosuppressive and chemotherapy agents.

Malignant diseases may also be associated with a bleeding tendency due to dysfunction of the coagulation pathway or impaired platelet synthesis in the bone marrow, as seen in patients with leukemia or bone metastases of solid tumors. A decrease in platelet count may occur as part of pancytopenia resulting from chemotherapy and, potentially, radiotherapy affecting the bone marrow. The use of hepatotoxic drugs can cause liver insufficiency, leading to splenomegaly and increased platelet sequestration. Additionally, the effects of malnutrition and the consequent deficiency of vitamin K, essential for the synthesis of vitamin K-dependent coagulation factors, must be considered.

Disseminated intravascular coagulation (DIC) can occur in malignant diseases, but it also occurs in sepsis, in pregnancy due to placental abruption following major

B. V. Bajkin (✉)
University of Novi Sad, Faculty of Medicine, Dentistry Clinic of Vojvodina, Novi Sad, Serbia
e-mail: branislav.bajkin@mf.uns.ac.rs

I. Urosevic
University of Novi Sad, Faculty of Medicine, University Clinical Center of Vojvodina, Clinic of Hematology, Novi Sad, Serbia

B. V. Bajkin (ed.), *Bleeding Disorders and Dentistry*,
https://doi.org/10.1007/978-3-032-26713-9_16

trauma and surgical procedures, and in many other conditions [2, 3]. DIC is a clinical-pathological syndrome characterized by hypercoagulability of the blood and the formation of numerous thrombi, which, on the one hand, cause ischemia in multiple organs and, on the other hand, lead to consumptive coagulopathy and a hemorrhagic syndrome. The underlying pathology involves uncontrolled thrombin generation due to blood contact with elevated levels of tissue factor, which, along with suppression of anticoagulant mechanisms and abnormal fibrinolysis, results in the formation of multiple fibrin deposits within small and medium-sized blood vessels. Reduced blood flow causes multiple organ insufficiency. Due to consumption of coagulation factors and platelets, hemorrhagic syndrome and systemic bleeding may occur, which is further exacerbated by pathologically accelerated fibrinolysis [2, 3].

The clinical presentation of the disease is variable, with the main symptoms typically reflecting the underlying condition, multiorgan failure, hemodynamic complications, and systemic hemorrhagic syndrome. Bleeding may manifest at venipuncture sites, as petechiae or ecchymoses on the skin, or as hemorrhage from the gastrointestinal tract, lungs, or central nervous system [2, 3]. A possible cutaneous manifestation of DIC is *purpura fulminans* (see Sect 7.1.3). The diagnosis is based on clinical presentation and laboratory parameters, primarily prolonged prothrombin time (PT), activated partial thromboplastin time (aPTT), thrombin time (TT), low platelet count, the appearance of schistocytes (fragmented erythrocytes) in the peripheral blood, low fibrinogen, and elevated fibrin degradation products (D-dimer) [2].

The mortality rate in DIC is approximately 30–80% [2]. Treatment primarily focuses on addressing the underlying disease that caused DIC and on controlling hemodynamic parameters. To prevent and control bleeding, fresh frozen plasma (FFP) and platelet concentrate are used. Cryoprecipitate can be administered when fibrinogen levels are low. In cases of pronounced fibrinolysis, antifibrinolytic agents can be included in the treatment, but caution is required because of the risk of thrombosis.

References

1. Idle M, Claiborne S, Patel K, Kademani D. Malignancy and haemostasis. In: Szumita RP, Szumita PM, editors. Hemostasis in dentistry. Springer eBook; 2018. p. 61–71.
2. Arruda VR, High KA. Coagulation disorders. In: Harrison's principles of internal medicine. 20th ed. McGraw-Hill Education eBook; 2018. p. 830–8.
3. Scully C. Haemathology. In: Scully's medical problems in dentistry. 7th ed. Elsevier: Churchill Livingstone; 2014. p. 212–75.

Dental Management of Patients with Malignancies Related to Hemostasis

17

Branislav V. Bajkin and Alison Dougall

Box 17.1 Dental Management of Patients with Malignancies

Dental considerations before the initiation of cancer therapy

- Provide the patient with oral hygiene instructions
- Get rid of all oral diseases that may exacerbate during cancer therapy
- If indicated, tooth extraction should be performed at least 7 days before initiation of chemotherapy, or at least 2 weeks before initiation of head and neck radiation therapy

Dental considerations during cancer therapy

- Early diagnosis and management of complications of radiation therapy and chemotherapy (mucositis, gingival bleeding, oral ulcerations, infections, taste alteration, xerostomia, radiation caries, hypersensitivity teeth, pulpal pain, osteoradionecrosis, muscular dysfunction)

Dental considerations after cancer therapy

- Recall appointments and treatment of cancer therapy sequelae

Oral surgery in patients with malignancy

- Consultation with the patient's oncologist
- Inpatient or outpatient treatment depending on the risk of the procedure

(continued)

B. V. Bajkin (✉)
University of Novi Sad, Faculty of Medicine, Dentistry Clinic of Vojvodina, Novi Sad, Serbia
e-mail: branislav.bajkin@mf.uns.ac.rs

A. Dougall
School of Dental Science, Trinity College Dublin, Dublin Dental University Hospital, Dublin, Ireland

B. V. Bajkin (ed.), *Bleeding Disorders and Dentistry*,
https://doi.org/10.1007/978-3-032-26713-9_17

Box 17.1 (continued)

- Preoperative laboratory testing should include a routine complete blood count and hemoglobin and hematocrit values to identify anemia
- In a patient with severe (hemoglobin levels <8 g/dl) or symptomatic anemia who requires extensive surgery when extensive blood loss is expected, blood transfusion is recommended
- In a patient with neutrophil count <1.000–2.000/mm^3, antibiotic prophylaxis is recommended
- In a patient with radiation therapy in the head and neck region, antibiotic prophylaxis is recommended for prevention of osteoradionecrosis
- Preoperative hemostatic laboratory screening (platelet count, prothrombin time, activated partial thromboplastin time, and bleeding time)
- Consider preoperative hematological treatment with fresh frozen plasma or platelet transfusion depending on the extensiveness of surgery and laboratory findings (INR >3; platelet count <30 × 10^9/L)[a]
- Choose the right time for elective surgery based on patients' general health and the phase of therapeutic treatment
- Minimize tissue trauma and blood loss (multiple visits may be necessary)
- In case of multiple tooth extractions, consider quadrant oral surgery to minimize trauma
- Use of local hemostatic agents and measures to control oral bleeding
- Provide a patient with postoperative instructions (avoid aspirin and other NSAIDs, soft and cold diet, phone number in case of an emergency) and regular follow-up

NSAIDs nonsteroidal anti-inflammatory drugs

[a]There is no general consensus regarding preoperative hematological treatment

Before any invasive dental intervention in patients with malignant disease, consultation with the attending oncologist is mandatory. Dental management of these patients requires careful planning based on thorough medical history, radiographic diagnostics, and the patient's overall medical condition. Data from medical records should include the type of malignancy, the extent of disease spread, and the treatment modalities used, which may include surgery, radiotherapy, chemotherapy, and immunotherapy. Dental management largely depends on the type of therapy and the treatment phase the patient is in (pretherapy, active treatment, or posttherapy) [1].

Chemotherapy data are critical, as not all drugs exert the same degree of immunosuppressive effect on the bone marrow. The medical history must include questions about spontaneous bleeding and bleeding during any previous surgery or trauma. Before oral surgical procedures, laboratory analyses, including a complete blood count (CBC) and assessment of hemostasis with a standard set of laboratory tests (prothrombin time [PT], activated partial thromboplastin time [aPTT], and platelet count), are necessary. For dental extraction, an INR of less than 3.5 is recommended. Platelet count is not a good predictor of postoperative bleeding risk. A platelet count greater than 30×10^9/L (or, according to other authors, greater than 50×10^9/L) is considered the minimum required for tooth extraction (see Chap. 8). Based on laboratory findings and the extent of the planned procedure, the need for prophylactic administration of fresh frozen plasma (FFP) or platelet concentrate is assessed. The procedure should be performed with minimal trauma and the use of local hemostatic agents and measures. For more extensive procedures, such as the extraction of multiple teeth, the procedure may be performed in a hospital setting or in multiple visits.

Routine preoperative CBC testing includes red blood cell count, hemoglobin level, hematocrit, and total and differential white blood cell counts, which may reveal anemia or leukopenia. Preoperative correction of anemia or antibiotic prophylaxis for leukopenia may be necessary. The timing of dental procedures should be chosen based on the patient's general health status and ongoing therapy. All patients with malignant diseases should undergo a complete dental examination before the initiation of radiotherapy or chemotherapy. All oral diseases that may worsen during cancer therapy should be ruled out, and nonrestorable teeth with poor prognosis, acute infection, or severe periodontal disease should be extracted [1]. Pretreatment care should also include oral hygiene instructions and tooth scaling and prophylaxis. Oral surgical procedures performed after the initiation of chemotherapy can lead to more frequent complications, such as bleeding, infection, or delayed wound healing [2]. Special caution is required during dental management in patients with malignant disease who have undergone head and neck radiotherapy, due to the risk of osteoradionecrosis, and in patients treated with antiresorptive drugs, such as bisphosphonates and denosumab, due to the risk of medication-related osteonecrosis of the jaws [3].

References

1. Little JW, Miller CS, Rhodus NL. Cancer and oral care of patients with cancer. In: Little and Falace's sdental management of the medically compromised patient. 9th ed. St. Louis: Elsevier; 2018. p. 480–514.
2. Akashi M, Kishimoto M, Kusumoto J, Yakushijin K, Matsuoka H, Komori T. Delayed socket healing after dental extraction in patients undergoing myelosuppressive chemotherapy for hematological malignancy: incidence and risk factors. J Oral Maxillofac Surg. 2018;76(10):2057–65.
3. Ruggiero SL, Dodson TB, Aghaloo T, Carlson ER, Ward BB, Kademani D. American Association of Oral and Maxillofacial Surgeons' position paper on medication-related osteonecrosis of the jaws-2022 update. J Oral Maxillofac Surg. 2022;80(5):920–43.

Part V

Antithrombotic Drugs

Dental Management of Patients Taking Antithrombotic Medications: General Considerations

18

Branislav V. Bajkin and Alison Dougall

Antithrombotic drugs can be classified into anticoagulants, antiplatelet drugs, and fibrinolytics (Fig. 18.1). Anticoagulant drugs, as their name implies, prevent blood coagulation and can be further classified into parenteral drugs (heparin and heparin derivatives) and oral anticoagulant drugs (vitamin K antagonists (VKAs) and direct oral anticoagulants (DOACs)). These medications are primarily used for preventive

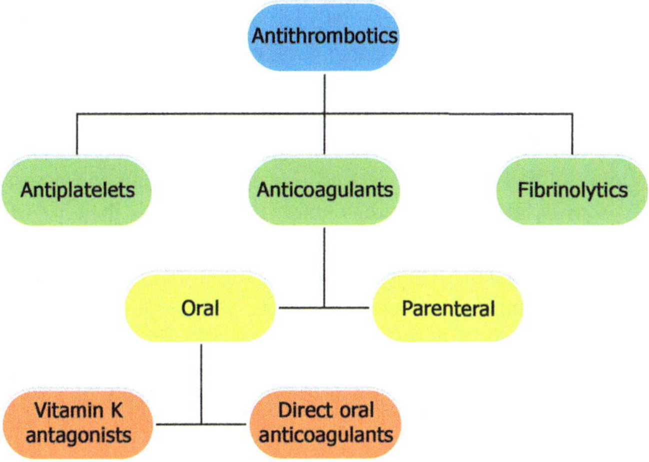

Fig. 18.1 Antithrombotic drugs

B. V. Bajkin (✉)
University of Novi Sad, Faculty of Medicine, Dentistry Clinic of Vojvodina, Novi Sad, Serbia
e-mail: branislav.bajkin@mf.uns.ac.rs

A. Dougall
School of Dental Science, Trinity College Dublin, Dublin Dental University Hospital, Dublin, Ireland

B. V. Bajkin (ed.), *Bleeding Disorders and Dentistry*,
https://doi.org/10.1007/978-3-032-26713-9_18

and therapeutic purposes in patients at risk of venous thromboembolism. Anticoagulant drugs, with the exception of certain DOACs, primarily reduce thrombin activity, either by inhibiting its synthesis or diminishing its functional activity. The main indications for anticoagulant drugs include venous thrombosis and/or pulmonary thromboembolism, atrial fibrillation, prosthetic heart valves, and following fractures of the lower extremities or hip surgery. Antiplatelet drugs affect platelet function, primarily by preventing platelet adhesion or aggregation. These agents are primarily used in the prevention and treatment of ischemic cardiovascular and cerebrovascular diseases. Given the prevalence of arterial and venous thrombosis in the general population, anticoagulant and antiplatelet drugs are among the most frequently prescribed pharmaceuticals.

Fibrinolytics or thrombolytics are drugs used in urgent clinical settings to dissolve thrombus and restore patency of occluded blood vessels, thereby enabling organ reperfusion. These drugs are administered systemically or delivered directly to the site of vascular occlusion via catheter. Common indications for their use include acute myocardial infarction, acute ischemic stroke, and massive pulmonary embolism. These drugs work by converting plasminogen into plasmin, an active enzyme that mediates fibrinolysis. This group of drugs includes streptokinase, anistreplase, urokinase, alteplase (recombinant tissue-type plasminogen activator, rtPA), reteplase, and tenecteplase [1]. Because fibrinolytic therapy is indicated in emergency situations and is short term, the use of these drugs is not of significant relevance to dental practice and therefore will not be discussed in the following text.

Oral surgical procedures in patients taking anticoagulant or antiplatelet therapy pose a significant clinical challenge. Continuous therapy may be associated with increased and prolonged bleeding during and after surgery. Conversely, any interruption of therapy increases the risk of thromboembolic complications. Successful dental treatment of these patients depends on understanding and assessing the risk of thrombosis associated with therapy interruption versus the risk of bleeding if therapy is continued.

In addition to antiplatelet therapy, several other factors influence the risk of bleeding, the most significant of which include comorbidities, concomitant medications that affect hemostatic function, and the degree of surgical trauma. Comorbidities must be considered when assessing the risk of postoperative bleeding. Liver and kidney diseases, hematologic malignancies, and congenital or acquired coagulopathies are among the conditions that may increase the risk of postoperative bleeding. It is reasonable to assume that the combined use of anticoagulant and antiplatelet therapy, as well as dual antiplatelet therapy, increases the risk of postoperative bleeding. In addition to the direct interaction of certain agents with anticoagulant or antiplatelet therapy, some drugs may increase the tendency toward bleeding through other mechanisms. A large number of medications, including immunosuppressive agents, nonsteroidal anti-inflammatory drugs (NSAIDs), and selective serotonin reuptake inhibitors, can affect either the platelet count or function.

When assessing the risk of bleeding, it is essential to consider the duration of the antithrombotic drug's effect, the need for regular monitoring of its activity, and whether there is a specific antidote for the medication the patient is receiving

(Table 18.1). For drugs with a short duration of action, such as heparin, omitting a single dose may be sufficient to prevent or manage postoperative bleeding. By contrast, VKAs and aspirin have effects that last for several days, and skipping a single dose usually does not significantly reduce the risk of postoperative bleeding. The availability of a specific antidote allows the drug's effects to be rapidly reversed, which can be crucial in cases of severe bleeding.

The risk of postoperative bleeding depends on the type of dental procedure and the degree of surgical trauma. Dental procedures that are unlikely to cause postoperative bleeding in patients receiving anticoagulant or antiplatelet therapy include local anesthesia, including inferior alveolar nerve block (IANB); supragingival removal of plaque and calculus; conservative tooth restoration; root canal treatment; taking impressions; and other prosthodontic and orthodontic procedures [2]. Except for tooth extraction, the literature lacks clear guidelines on the safety and assessment of postoperative bleeding risk for other oral surgical procedures. Most researchers suggest that extracting up to three teeth is considered a moderate-bleeding-risk procedure, while extracting more than three teeth, procedures that require raising a mucoperiosteal flap, or biopsies should be considered higher-risk procedures for postoperative bleeding [2–4]. In addition to the extent of the procedure, it is necessary to consider the anatomical region of the oral surgery, the degree of tissue inflammation, and the availability and applicability of local hemostatic agents and measures. Dental procedures in highly vascularized areas, as well as those on the floor of the mouth with potential airway obstruction in case of bleeding, should be considered high-risk procedures. Periodontal surgery, as well as surgical procedures performed in inflamed tissue, are also associated with a higher risk of postoperative bleeding.

Table 18.1 Duration, monitoring, and reversal agents for antithrombotic drugs

Drug	Approximate duration of the effect[a]	Routine monitoring	Antidote
Heparin	6 h	aPTT 1.5–2.5 times None for low-dose therapy	Protamine sulfate
LMWHs	Up to 24 h	None	No antidote; protamine sulfate has limited effectiveness
Fondaparinux	24 h	None	No antidote
Warfarin	2–5 days	INR 2.0–3.5	Vitamin K
Acenocoumarol	2 days	INR 2.0–3.5	Vitamin K
Dabigatran	22 h	None	Idarucizumab
Rivaroxaban	24 h	None	Andexanet alfa
Apixaban	24 h	None	Andexanet alfa

[a]The duration of the drug's effect is shown only as an orientation because it can depend on numerous factors (e.g., the route heparin administration and the doses used, the applied LMWH preparation, individual response and diet in the case of vitamin K antagonists, kidney function in patients on dabigatran therapy, as well as many other factors)

LMWHs low-molecular-weight heparins, *INR* International Normalized Ratio, *aPTT* activated partial thromboplastin time

Discontinuation of antithrombotic therapy increases the risk of thromboembolic events. Identifying and assessing thromboembolism risk factors do not fall within the primary domain of dental professionals. However, dentists, primarily oral and maxillofacial surgeons, should be members of a multidisciplinary team and involved in the decision-making process to ensure the safest possible management of these patients during surgical procedures. A basic understanding of key thromboembolic risk factors is therefore essential. The risk of a thromboembolic event during therapy interruption varies among patients. This risk must be thoroughly assessed when planning a procedure with temporary cessation of antithrombotic therapy or bridging treatment with heparin or heparin-derived agents. The risk of thromboembolic events primarily depends on the underlying condition necessitating anticoagulant or antiplatelet therapy, but it is also influenced by other factors.

If available, established scoring systems should be used to assess thromboembolic risk. The most commonly used scoring systems for atrial fibrillation are $CHADS_2$ and $CHADS_2$-VASc [5]. The $CHADS_2$-VASc scoring system is an extension of the $CHADS_2$ score that, in addition to congestive heart failure, hypertension, age ≥ 75 years, diabetes mellitus, and previous stroke, also includes vascular disease in patients aged 65–74 years and the patient's sex as risk factors. $CHADS_2$-VASc scores of ≥ 2 indicate the need for anticoagulant therapy [6], whereas patients with a score of 0 or 1 may be managed with aspirin therapy [5]. Atrial fibrillation is one of the most common indications for anticoagulant treatment with VKAs or DOACs. The most serious complication of atrial fibrillation is thromboembolism, i.e., ischemic cerebrovascular stroke [5, 7].

Risk factors for venous thrombosis include venous stasis, a hypercoagulable state, and blood vessel injury. Anticoagulant therapy duration depends on the presence of one or more risk factors for venous thrombosis, the underlying cause, and whether it is accompanied by pulmonary thromboembolism. Therapy can last for several months or be lifelong. A hypercoagulable state is usually diagnosed after a thromboembolic event. These conditions cause venous thromboembolism far more often than arterial thromboembolism. They can be congenital or acquired. The most common inherited hypercoagulable states are protein C and S deficiencies, the factor V Leiden mutation, and antithrombin deficiency. Acquired hypercoagulable states include antiphospholipid syndrome, malignancies, myeloproliferative disorders, and heparin-induced thrombocytopenia (HIT) [5]. Conditions associated with recurrent thrombosis and a high risk of thromboembolism, such as antithrombin deficiency and antiphospholipid syndrome, require long-term, sometimes lifelong use of oral anticoagulant therapy [8].

Heart valves may be dysfunctional due to stenosis or regurgitation. Surgical interventions on heart valves include repair or replacement of the insufficient valve. Following reparative heart valve procedures, antithrombotic therapy is administered. Patients with prosthetic heart valves have a high risk of thromboembolism. However, within this group, the risk varies depending on the type and position of the replaced valve. For instance, biological valves are less thrombogenic than mechanical valves, which are more durable. Caged-ball mechanical prosthetic valves are more thrombogenic than bileaflet valves. Additionally, a prosthetic valve in the mitral position has an increased risk of thromboembolic complications compared to those placed in the aortic position. Depending on the position of the biological prosthetic valve, either antiplatelet or oral anticoagulant therapy may be indicated. Mechanical heart valves in any position require VKA therapy [5]. In general, the risk of thromboembolism is higher with older-generation heart valves and with valves in the mitral position compared to newer-generation heart valves and those in the aortic position.

According to the recommendation of the American College of Chest Physicians [9], all patients receiving oral anticoagulant therapy can be classified as high, moderate, or low risk for thromboembolism upon discontinuation of therapy without heparin bridging. Patients at high risk have an annual thromboembolism risk greater than 10%; moderate-risk patients have a risk between 5% and 10%; and low-risk patients have an annual risk less than 5%. Patients and conditions associated with a high risk of thromboembolism during temporary cessation of anticoagulant therapy include the following [9]:

1. For patients with mechanical heart valves—valve in the mitral position, older-generation mechanical heart valves in the aortic position with higher thrombogenicity (caged ball, tilting disc), and ischemic stroke or transient ischemic attack in the last 6 months
2. For patients with atrial fibrillation—$CHADS_2$ score of 5 or 6, ischemic stroke or transient ischemic attack in the last 3 months, and rheumatic heart valve disease
3. For patients with venous thromboembolism—venous thromboembolism in the last 3 months and severe thrombophilia (for instance, protein C and S deficiency, antithrombin deficiency, antiphospholipid syndrome, or multiple risk factors for thromboembolism)

Ischemic cardiovascular and cerebrovascular diseases are among the leading causes of mortality in developed countries. Risk factors for these diseases are numerous, and the most significant include hypertension, hyperlipidemia, diabetes mellitus, obesity, physical inactivity, a diet rich in saturated fatty acids, smoking, and a positive family history. Coronary artery disease can be classified as stable (stable angina pectoris) or unstable (unstable angina pectoris and myocardial infarction). Antiplatelet therapy is used for both primary and secondary prevention of these diseases. Aspirin is by far the most commonly used antiplatelet drug, administered in doses ranging from 81 to 325 mg for cardiovascular prophylaxis. Aspirin is used in primary prophylaxis, and aspirin monotherapy remains the standard of care for patients who have undergone myocardial revascularization by coronary artery bypass grafting [10]. Following percutaneous coronary intervention, dual antiplatelet therapy, most commonly with aspirin and clopidogrel, is indicated [11]. Due to the risk of thrombosis, dual antiplatelet therapy should not be discontinued for any surgery for at least 6 weeks after placement of a bare-metal stent or for at least 6 months after placement of a drug-eluting stent [9]. Simultaneous use of aspirin and clopidogrel increases the risk of bleeding, but premature discontinuation of either of these two drugs has been identified as a major risk factor for stent thrombosis [12].

Ischemic cerebrovascular diseases (ischemic stroke and transient ischemic attack) usually require antiplatelet therapy. Treatment of ischemic stroke caused by atrial fibrillation follows recommendations for this disease [5]. Acute ischemic stroke is classified according to the Trial of Org 10172 in Acute Stroke Treatment (TOAST) into five categories: (1) large-artery atherosclerosis, (2) cardioembolism, (3) small-artery occlusion, (4) stroke of other determined etiology, and (5) stroke of undetermined etiology [13]. The clinical manifestations of acute ischemic stroke depend on the affected blood vessel and the corresponding brain region. Recent myocardial infarction, cerebrovascular stroke, and transient ischemic attack are risk factors for recurrence of the same complication if antithrombotic therapy is discontinued.

Given the frequency of oral surgical procedures and the growing number of patients receiving anticoagulant and antiplatelet therapy, dentists must be familiar with the mechanisms of action of these drugs, their interactions with medications commonly used in dental practice, the prevention and management of postoperative bleeding complications, and current recommendations for the dental management of these patients. Despite numerous studies published in recent years supporting the safety of oral surgical procedures, particularly tooth extractions, in patients receiving anticoagulant and antiplatelet therapy, there remain doubts and disagreements in everyday dental clinical practice [14].

Oral surgical procedures in patients receiving anticoagulant or antiplatelet therapy require consultation with the patient's physician. The dentist should inform the patient that, according to current guidelines, interruption of anticoagulant or antiplatelet therapy is generally not recommended for most oral surgical procedures [14]. If the therapy is interrupted for any reason, this should never be based on the dentist's recommendation, but rather on the advice of the physician who prescribed the treatment.

References

1. Weitz JI. Antiplatelet, anticoagulant, and fibrinolytic drugs in section disorders of hemostasis. In: Harrison's principles of internal medicine. 20th ed. McGraw-Hill Education eBook; 2018. p. 843–58.
2. Scottish Dental Clinical Effectiveness Programme. Management of dental patients taking anticoagulants or antiplatelet drugs. Dental clinical guidance. 2rd ed. 2022. Available online at: https://www.sdcep.org.uk/media/ypnl2cpz/sdcep-management-of-dental-patients-taking-anticoagulants-or-antiplatelet-drugs-2nd-edition.pdf. Accessed Feb 2024.
3. Bajkin BV, Vujkov SB, Milekic BR, Vuckovic BA. Risk factors for bleeding after oral surgery in patients who continued using oral anticoagulant therapy. J Am Dent Assoc. 2015;146(6):375–81.
4. Broekema FI, Minnen B, Jansma J, Bos RR. Risk of bleeding after dentoalveolar surgery in patients taking anticoagulants. Br J Oral Maxillofac Surg. 2014;52(3):e15–9.
5. Hohlfelder B. Stratifying thromboembolic risk: why is your patient on antithrombotic medications? In: Szumita RP, Szumita PM, editors. Hemostasis in dentistry. Cham: Springer; 2018. p. 73–89.

6. Kirchhof P, Benussi S, Kotecha D, Ahlsson A, Altar D, Casadei B, et al. ESC guidelines for the management of atrial fibrillation. Eur Heart J. 2016;37(38):2893–962.
7. Chugh SS, Havmoeller R, Narayanan K, Singh D, Rienstra M, Benjamin EJ, et al. Worldwide epidemiology of atrial fibrillation: a global burden of disease 2010 study. Circulation. 2014;129(8):837–47.
8. Ansell J, Hirsh J, Hylek E, Jacobson A, Crowther M, Palareti G, American College of Chest Physicians. Pharmacology and management of the vitamin K antagonists: American College of Chest Physicians Evidence-Based Clinical Practice Guidelines (8th Edition). Chest. 2008;133(6 Suppl):160S–98S.
9. Douketis JD, Spyropoulos AC, Spencer FA, Mayr M, Jaffer AK, Eckman MH, et al. Perioperative management of antithrombotic therapy: antithrombotic therapy and prevention of thrombosis. 9th ed. American College of Chest Physicians Evidence-Based Clinical Practice Guidelines. Chest. 2012;141(2 Suppl):e326S–50S.
10. Kulik A, Ruel M, Jneid H, Ferguson TB, Hiratzka LF, Ikonomidis JS, et al. Secondary prevention after coronary artery bypass graft surgery: a scientific statement from the American Heart Association. Circulation. 2015;131(10):927–64.
11. Levine GN, Bates ER, Bittl JA, Brindis RG, Fihn SD, Fleisher LA, et al. 2016 ACC/AHA guideline focused update on duration of dual antiplatelet therapy in patients with coronary artery disease: a report of the American College of Cardilogy/American Heart Association Task Force on clinical practice guidelines. J Am Coll Cardiol. 2016;68(10):1082–115.
12. Grines CL, Bonow RO, Casey DE Jr, Gardner TJ, Lockhart PB, Moliterno DJ, et al. Prevention of premature discontinuation of dual antiplatelet therapy in patients with coronary artery stents: a science advisory from the American Heart Association, American College of Cardiology, Society for Cardiovascular Angiography and Interventions, American College of Surgeons, and American Dental Association, with representation from the American College of Physicians. Circulation. 2007;115(6):813–8.
13. Adams HP Jr, Bendixen BH, Kappelle LJ, Biller J, Love BB, Gordon DL, et al. Classification of subtype of acute ischemic stroke. Definitions for use in a multicenter clinical trial. TOAST. Trial of org 10172 in acute stroke treatment. Stroke. 1993;24:35–41.
14. Wahl MJ, Miller CS, Rhodus NL, Kämmerer P, Dinkova A, Lalla RV, Bajkin BV. Anticoagulants are dental friendly. Oral Surg Oral Med Oral Pathol Oral Radiol. 2018;125(2):103–6.

19 Parenteral Anticoagulant Drugs

Branislav V. Bajkin and Ivana Urosevic

Parenteral anticoagulant agents include unfractionated heparin (UFH), low-molecular-weight heparins (LMWHs), synthetic heparin analogs, danaparoid sodium, and parenteral direct thrombin inhibitors (lepirudin, desirudin, bivalirudin, and argatroban) (Table 19.1). Parenteral direct thrombin inhibitors, along with danaparoid, are used as alternatives in patients with heparin-induced thrombocytopenia (HIT) for the treatment of deep vein thrombosis and during orthopedic surgical procedures. These drugs are primarily used in hospital settings and will not be discussed further in the text.

Table 19.1 Parenteral anticoagulant drugs

Heparins	Direct thrombin inhibitors
Unfractionated heparin	Recombinant hirudins
Low-molecular-weight heparins	Lepirudin
Dalteparin	Desirudin
Enoxaparin sodium	Bivalirudin
Nadroparin calcium	Argatroban
Tinzaparin	
Ardeparin	
Reviparin	
Synthetic heparins	
Fondaparinux	
Idraparinux	
Heparinoid	
Danaparoid sodium	

B. V. Bajkin (✉)
University of Novi Sad, Faculty of Medicine, Dentistry Clinic of Vojvodina, Novi Sad, Serbia
e-mail: branislav.bajkin@mf.uns.ac.rs

I. Urosevic
University of Novi Sad, Faculty of Medicine, University Clinical Center of Vojvodina, Clinic of Hematology, Novi Sad, Serbia

B. V. Bajkin (ed.), *Bleeding Disorders and Dentistry*,
https://doi.org/10.1007/978-3-032-26713-9_19

19.1 Heparin

Heparin is a natural anticoagulant. Chemically, it is a sulfated glycosaminoglycan with numerous sulfate groups that make it highly negatively charged. It was originally isolated from the liver, which is reflected in its name. Heparin is synthesized in the secretory granules of mast cells and basophilic blood cells. Its concentration in the bloodstream is low, but when administered for therapeutic purposes, it exhibits a potent anticoagulant effect with an almost immediate onset of action.

The effect of heparin on the hemostatic mechanism is complex. Its effect is predominantly indirect, mediated by its binding to antithrombin (AT, formerly known as antithrombin III), which enhances AT activity by up to a thousandfold [1]. AT is a natural inhibitor of coagulation proteases, primarily thrombin and FXa, but also others (FIXa, FXIa, and FXIIa). Heparin not only affects platelet function by enhancing aggregation but is also a potent inhibitor of platelet activation induced by thrombin [2–4].

Heparin is the most commonly used parenteral anticoagulant. Heparins are classified by molecular weight into high- and low-molecular-weight forms. Synthetic heparin derivatives (such as fondaparinux) are also available. The main indications for heparin use include the treatment of deep vein thrombosis and pulmonary embolism, the prevention of deep vein thrombosis (such as following orthopedic surgical procedures on the lower extremities), use in acute coronary syndrome, and use in patients undergoing hemodialysis.

Unfractionated Heparin

UFH is a heterogeneous mixture of polysaccharide chains with molecular weights ranging from 3000 to 30,000 Daltons (Da), with an average molecular weight of approximately 15,000 Da [2, 5]. Commercial agents are of animal origin and are primarily derived from intestinal mucosa. They inhibit thrombin and FXa equally, but thrombin is significantly more sensitive to the effect of the heparin/AT complex. Thrombin inhibition is achieved through formation of a heparin/AT/thrombin complex, which requires the presence of long heparin chains [2]. It is administered exclusively via the parenteral route, either intravenously or subcutaneously. For therapeutic purposes, it is primarily administered intravenously because of unpredictable bioavailability following subcutaneous administration. For this reason, subcutaneous doses are typically higher than intravenous doses.

After intravenous UFH administration, the effect is almost instantaneous, within a few minutes. UFH dosing is based on the patient's body weight, clinical indication for treatment, and relevant laboratory parameters, including activated partial thromboplastin time (aPTT) and anti-FXa activity. Treatment is usually initiated with an intravenous bolus of 5000 units or 70–100 units/kg, followed by a continuous intravenous infusion at 12–20 units/kg/h [5–7]. Higher doses are recommended for venous thromboembolism than for acute coronary syndrome [2]. The drug has a short, dose-dependent half-life that typically ranges from 1 to 2 h [2–6, 8, 9]. UFH is typically administered as a continuous intravenous infusion in a hospital setting, with frequent monitoring of aPTT. In patients undergoing hemodialysis, UFH is administered intravenously in an outpatient setting.

The anticoagulant effect of UFH is neutralized by binding to endothelium and plasma proteins. A smaller fraction of the drug is eliminated by renal excretion. Dose-dependent clearance of UFH is primarily explained by endothelial binding, while variable plasma protein binding among individuals accounts for the variability in its anticoagulant effect [5]. Therefore, careful laboratory monitoring and frequent dose adjustments are necessary. A prolonged aPTT of 1.5–2.5 times control is considered the therapeutic range [2–4, 6, 8, 9]. aPTT should be tested every 4–6 h following UFH bolus administration. Assessment of anti-factor Xa activity is an alternative to aPTT measurement for monitoring UFH therapy. The therapeutic range is 0.3–0.7 anti-Xa units/mL [2, 5, 6].

Although UFH can also be administered subcutaneously, its bioavailability via this route is significantly lower, and the effect is less predictable. Only a small number of patients have aPTT values within the recommended therapeutic range after subcutaneous administration [2, 10]. This suggests that subcutaneous administration of UFH should be reserved for patients at low thromboembolic risk [11] or that high doses may be required to overcome the reduced bioavailability associated with this route [2, 5]. For prophylaxis, a fixed dose of 5000 units of UFH is typically administered subcutaneously, two to three times a day [5–7]. During prophylactic use, routine monitoring of the anticoagulant effect is typically not required.

UFH is used for both the prevention and treatment of acute venous thrombosis and pulmonary embolism. In cases requiring urgent initiation of anticoagulant therapy, treatment typically begins with heparin and a few days later is followed by the concurrent introduction of oral anticoagulant therapy with vitamin K antagonists (VKAs), whose therapeutic effect develops significantly more slowly. After achieving a stable therapeutic effect with oral anticoagulant therapy, heparin is discontinued. The duration of concurrent heparin and VKA administration depends on the rate at which the therapeutic effect of oral anticoagulant therapy is achieved. Heparin is also used prophylactically in patients at high risk of thromboembolism in whom oral anticoagulant therapy is temporarily discontinued due to major surgical intervention (bridging therapy).

The main adverse effect of heparin is bleeding, which can occur at the surgical site or elsewhere in the body. When administering UFH intravenously, strict adherence to protocol is necessary to achieve the appropriate therapeutic effect with minimal risk of bleeding. Due to the drug's short half-life, withholding the next dose is usually sufficient in cases of bleeding. Serious bleeding complications require the administration of protamine sulfate, the antidote to heparin (Table 18.1). Protamine sulfate is administered intravenously, and 1 mg of the drug neutralizes approximately 100 units of heparin [2, 5]. In addition to bleeding, other adverse reactions include thrombocytopenia, osteoporosis, elevated transaminase levels, allergic reactions, and adverse skin reactions. Heparin resistance may also occur, necessitating the use of higher doses of the drug to achieve the therapeutic effect.

A serious complication that may occur following administration of this drug is heparin-induced thrombocytopenia (HIT). It typically develops between 5 and 10 days after initiation of therapy (see Sect. 7.1.5). HIT occurs in approximately 0.1–5% of patients treated with heparin [12] and may be accompanied by paradoxical thrombosis. This so-called white clot syndrome is immune-mediated and not dose-dependent.

Low-Molecular-Weight Heparins

LMWHs are obtained by chemical or enzymatic depolymerization of high-molecular-weight heparin into fragments with significantly lower molecular weight, averaging 4000–5000 Da (range, 2000–9000 Da) [2, 5]. Low-molecular-weight fragments exhibit reduced affinity for plasma proteins and cellular components, which underlies the differences in pharmacokinetics and mechanisms of action between LMWHs and UFH. Additionally, because of differences in the methods used, various LMWH preparations exhibit distinct pharmacokinetic and pharmacodynamic profiles.

The mechanism of action of LMWHs is similar to that of UFH, as they also act as a catalyst for AT, but they exhibit significantly greater activity against FXa than against thrombin. This is because the shorter chains of LMWHs cannot bind simultaneously to both AT and thrombin. The anti-FXa to anti-FIIa activity ratio ranges from 2:1 to 4:1, depending on the LMWH preparation used [2, 8]. LMWHs have several advantages over UFH, including greater bioavailability, a longer half-life, and a more predictable and consistent anticoagulant effect due to reduced binding to plasma proteins, macrophages, and endothelial cells. These properties enable subcutaneous administration of these drugs once or twice a day in an outpatient setting without the need for routine monitoring of drug effects.

LMWHs, including dalteparin, enoxaparin sodium, nadroparin calcium, tinzaparin, ardeparin, reviparin, and others, differ in molecular weight, pharmacokinetics, and antithrombotic activity, making direct comparison of efficacy difficult. Bioavailability of these drugs is approximately 90% after subcutaneous administration. They achieve maximal effect within 3–5 h, with a half-life of 3–6 h that is not dose-dependent [2]. Because of renal elimination, their half-life is prolonged in patients with renal insufficiency.

LMWHs are administered in fixed doses or at doses based on the patient's body weight. Prophylactic doses are typically 4000–5000 units once a day, or slightly lower if these drugs are administered twice a day. Dosing largely depends on the specific LMWH used. Anti-FXa activity can be used to assess the effect of these drugs. However, except in special circumstances, such as use during pregnancy, in obese patients, and in those with renal insufficiency, there is no need for routine monitoring of LMWH anticoagulant activity [2, 5, 8, 13]. The therapeutic range of anti-FXa activity is 0.5–1.2 units/mL, while the prophylactic range is slightly lower at 0.2–0.5 units/mL [5].

Indications for LMWHs are identical to those for UFH and primarily include the prevention of deep vein thrombosis and the treatment of acute venous thrombosis and pulmonary embolism. These drugs are also used in the treatment of acute coronary syndrome, for the prevention of graft thrombosis in vascular surgery, and prophylactically following major orthopedic surgery [2, 7, 13]. LMWHs are also used as bridging therapy in patients at risk of thromboembolism in whom oral anticoagulant therapy is temporarily discontinued due to major surgery.

The adverse effects of these drugs are similar to those that may occur with UFH, but their incidence is lower. The reduced incidence of bleeding following LMWH administration is attributed to the lesser effect of these drugs on platelets, endothelium, and von Willebrand factor (VWF) [2, 13], while the decreased incidence of HIT is a result of reduced affinity of these preparations for platelets [2, 3, 8]. Additionally, LMWHs less frequently cause osteoporosis than UFH [2]. Protamine sulfate is less effective as an antidote in patients undergoing LMWH therapy than in those receiving UFH therapy.

Fondaparinux

Fondaparinux is a synthetic analog of the low-molecular-weight AT-binding pentasaccharide sequence of heparin, with a molecular weight of 1700 Da. It is used for prophylaxis in patients at risk of thromboembolism and following orthopedic surgery. It can also be used instead of UFH or LMWHs as initial therapy for thromboembolism and in patients with acute coronary syndrome. Fondaparinux has an extremely high affinity for AT. Because of its low molecular weight, after binding to AT, it cannot form a complex with thrombin, exerting its effect only on FXa. Compared to UFH and LMWHs, it has several advantages: better bioavailability after subcutaneous administration, a longer half-life, and once-daily administration in fixed doses without the need for laboratory monitoring. Following subcutaneous administration, its bioavailability is nearly 100%, and its plasma half-life is approximately 17 h. For prophylactic purposes, it is administered at a dose of 2.5 mg. The therapeutic dose for venous thromboembolism and pulmonary embolism is 5–10 mg once a day, administered concomitantly with VKAs. It is completely excreted via the kidneys, and its clearance is not dose-dependent. Fondaparinux is contraindicated in patients with renal insufficiency. The primary adverse effect is bleeding, and there is no specific antidote for this drug. Because it does not bind to platelets, it does not cause HIT [5–7].

Danaparoid Sodium

Danaparoid sodium is a mixture of glycosaminoglycans (heparan sulfate, dermatan sulfate, and chondroitin sulfate) with anti-FXa activity. The half-life of this drug is approximately 25 h and there is no specific antidote. The drug is approved in some countries as an alternative to heparin in patients with HIT [2].

References

1. Hall JE, Hall ME. Hemostasis and blood coagulation. In: Guyton and Hall textbook of medical physiology. 14th ed. Philadelphia: Elsevier; 2021. p. 477–88.
2. Hirsh J, Bauer KA, Donati MB, Gould M, Samama MM, Weitz JI, American College of Chest Physicians. Parenteral anticoagulants: American College of Chest Physicians evidence-based clinical practice guidelines (8th Edition). Chest. 2008;133(6 Suppl):141S–59S.
3. Scully C, Wolff A. Oral surgery in patients on anticoagulant therapy. Oral Surg Oral Med Oral Pathol Oral Radiol Endod. 2002;94:57–64.
4. Scully C. Haemathology. In: Scully's medical problems in dentistry. 7th ed. Elsevier: Churchill Livingstone; 2014. p. 212–75.

5. Weitz JI. Antiplatelet, anticoagulant, and fibrinolytic drugs in section disorders of hemostasis. In: Harrison's principles of internal medicine. 20th ed. McGraw-Hill Education eBook; 2018. p. 843–58.
6. Bermudez P, Beushausen M, Horan MP. Management of inherited, acquired, and iatrogenically induced coagulopathies in oral surgery. In: A textbook of advanced oral and maxillofacial surgery, vol. 3. InTech; 2016. p. 175–210.
7. Reardon DP, Zemaitis C. Review of anticoagulants. In: Szumita RP, Szumita PM, editors. Hemostasis in dentistry. Springer eBook; 2018. p. 99–108.
8. Little JW, Miller CS, Henry RG, McIntosh BA. Antithrombotic agents: implications in dentistry. Oral Surg Oral Med Oral Pathol Oral Radiol Endod. 2002;93:544–51.
9. Mehra P, Cottrell DA, Bestgen SC, Booth DF. Management of heparin therapy in the high-risk, chronically anticoagulated, oral surgery patient: a review and a proposed nomogram. J Oral Maxillofac Surg. 2000;58:198–202.
10. Montalescot G, Polle V, Collet JP, Leprince P, Bellanger A, Gandjbakhch I, et al. Low-molecular-weight heparin after mechanical heart valve replacement. Circulation. 2001;101:1083–6.
11. Meurin P, Tabet JY. Can we use a low molecular weight heparin after mechanical prosthetic heart valve surgery? Heart. 2008;94:131–2.
12. Greinacher A, Warkentin TE, Chong BH. Heparin-induced thrombocytopenia. In section: disorders of platelet number and/or function. In: Michelson AD, Cattaneo M, Frelinger A, Newman PJ, editors. Platelets. 4th ed. Cambridge, MA: Academic Press; 2019. p. 741–67.
13. Schardt-Sacco D, Hill C. Update on coagulopathies. Oral Surg Oral Med Oral Pathol Oral Radiol Endod. 2000;90:559–63.

Oral Surgery in Patients Taking Heparin 20

Branislav V. Bajkin and Alison Dougall

Box 20.1 Dental Management of Patients Taking Heparin

Heparin

1. Unfractionated heparin (IV or SC route of administration)
2. Low-molecular-weight heparins (mostly SC route of administration; LMWHs have different pharmacokinetics)
3. Synthetized heparin analogue (fondaparinux)

Oral surgery in patients taking heparin

- Consult the patient's physician
- In a case of short-term heparin therapy, the procedure can be delayed until the end of treatment
- Minor oral surgery, including tooth extraction, is considered to be safe without stopping UFH or LMWHs
- Routine preoperative laboratory screening is usually not required
- For patients taking UFH IV in therapeutic doses, perioperative monitoring of the anticoagulant effect by aPTT or anti-FXa activity may be required
- Due to short life of heparin, the dose before surgery may be omitted in a case of more extensive surgery, but the risk of thromboembolism has to be estimated

(continued)

B. V. Bajkin (✉)
University of Novi Sad, Faculty of Medicine, Dentistry Clinic of Vojvodina, Novi Sad, Serbia
e-mail: branislav.bajkin@mf.uns.ac.rs

A. Dougall
School of Dental Science, Trinity College Dublin, Dublin Dental University Hospital, Dublin, Ireland

B. V. Bajkin (ed.), *Bleeding Disorders and Dentistry*,
https://doi.org/10.1007/978-3-032-26713-9_20

Box 20.1 (continued)

- In renal dialysis patients, oral surgery is best carried out on the day after dialysis. The effects of heparinization have then ceased
- In a patient taking VKA, bridging therapy with UFH or LMWHs is not recommended for minor oral surgery including tooth extraction. Major surgical procedures in patients with high risk of thromboembolism may require bridging therapy which should be initiated and carefully planned by patient's physicians
- Schedule a patient at the beginning of the work week
- Use of local anesthesia with vasoconstrictor
- Minimally traumatic surgical technique; multiple appointments may be necessary
- Use of local hemostatic agents and measures to control oral bleeding
- For pain relief, use acetaminophen if not contraindicated; avoid aspirin and other NSAIDs
- Provide a patient with postoperative instructions (soft and cold diet, phone number in case of an emergency) and regular follow-up

IV intravenous, *SC* subcutaneous, *UFH* unfractionated heparin, *LMWHs* low-molecular-weight heparins, *aPTT* activated partial thromboplastin time, *VKA* vitamin K antagonists, *NSAIDs* nonsteroidal anti-inflammatory drugs

Most of the data in the literature on the dental management of patients on heparin therapy come from studies assessing the safety of performing oral surgery when oral anticoagulant therapy is temporarily interrupted by bridging with low-molecular-weight heparins (LMWHs) to reduce the risk of postoperative bleeding. It is important to emphasize that studies have shown no need to bridge oral anticoagulant therapy with heparin for tooth extraction [1, 2]. If such an approach is suggested by the physician, or if the patient is receiving LMWH therapy for other reasons, oral surgical procedures can be safely performed without interrupting therapy, provided that appropriate local hemostatic measures are used [1–4].

Although not indicated for simple tooth extractions, bridging therapy with LMWHs or unfractionated heparin (UFH) may be beneficial during major oral or maxillofacial surgical procedures in patients receiving oral anticoagulant therapy. LMWHs are most frequently used for these purposes, while intravenous UFH may be indicated in patients with a high risk of thrombosis and in those treated in hospital settings. The decision to use bridging therapy is made by the attending physician, in consultation with the oral and maxillofacial surgeon, based on an assessment of the bleeding risk versus the risk of thromboembolism. It should be noted that the effect of UFH lasts up to 6 h following intravenous administration, whereas the effect of LMWHs can last for up to 24 h, depending on the specific preparation used [3, 5]. Bridging treatment, if indicated, can be complex and depends on numerous factors, including the risk of thrombosis (see Chap. 18), the type of surgery, the risk of intraoperative and postoperative bleeding, the presence of comorbidities, as well as other factors [5, 6]. The dentist/surgeon must be fully informed about the therapeutic plan, including the timing of discontinuation of oral anticoagulant therapy, the initiation of heparin prophylaxis, the need for temporary discontinuation of heparin immediately prior to the surgical procedure, the timing of postoperative reinitiation of heparin, and the subsequent reintroduction of oral anticoagulant therapy. With careful planning, the risk of bleeding, even in more extensive surgical procedures, can be minimized while ensuring maximum protection of the patient from thromboembolic complications.

UFH is typically administered intravenously over a shorter period of time and is used only for prolonged periods in patients undergoing dialysis. Oral surgery in these patients should be performed the day after dialysis. Thus, the effect of heparin, which has a short half-life, is avoided, and the procedure is performed at a time when toxic metabolites have been cleared from the circulation and the dialysis effect is maximal [3, 7, 8].

It is rare that oral surgical treatment is required in patients receiving continuous intravenous infusion of UFH. Usually, such a procedure can be postponed after the stabilization of the underlying disease and improvement in overall medical condition.

When tooth extraction must be performed while the patient is receiving intravenous UFH therapy, the procedure can be carried out safely following prior assessment of activated partial thromboplastin time (aPTT) and with the use of local hemostatic measures and agents [9].

References

1. Bajkin BV, Popovic SL, Selakovic SDj. Randomized, prospective trial comparing bridging therapy using low-molecular-weight heparin with maintenance of oral anticoagulation during extraction of teeth. J Oral Maxillofac Surg. 2009;67(5):990–5.
2. Erden İ, Çakcak Erden E, Aksu T, Gölcük ŞE, Turan B, Erkol A, Akçakoyun M, Sayın T. Comparison of uninterrupted warfarin and bridging therapy using low-molecular weight heparin with respect to the severity of bleeding after dental extractions in patients with prosthetic valves. Anatol J Cardiol. 2016;16(7):467–73.
3. Scully C. Haemathology. In: Scully's medical problems in dentistry. 7th ed. Elsevier: Churchill Livingstone; 2014. p. 212–75.
4. Little JW, Miller CS, Rhodus NL. Acquired bleeding and hypercoagulable disorders. In: Little and Falace's sdental management of the medically compromised patient. 9th ed. St. Louis: Elsevier; 2018. p. 428–56.
5. Rimsans J, Sylvester KW. Perioperative management of patients on anticoagulant medications: general principles in medicine and surgery. In: Szumita RP, Szumita PM, editors. Hemostasis in dentistry. Springer eBook; 2018. p. 143–50.
6. Mehra P, Cottrell DA, Bestgen SC, Booth DF. Management of heparin therapy in the high-risk, chronically anticoagulated, oral surgery patient: a review and a proposed nomogram. J Oral Maxillofac Surg. 2000;58:198–202.

7. Costantinides F, Castronovo G, Vettori E, Frattini C, Artero ML, Bevilacqua L, Berton F, Nicolin V, Di Lenarda R. Dental care for patients with end-stage renal disease and undergoing hemodialysis. Int J Dent. 2018;2018:9610892. eCollection 2018.
8. Pendem S, Lakshmi Narayana G, Ravi P. End stage renal disease: not a contraindication for minor oral surgery-protocol for the management of oral Surgery patients with ESRD on hemodialysis. J Maxillofac Oral Surg. 2017;16(2):231–7.
9. Morimoto Y, Niwa H, Minematsu K. Risk factors affecting hemorrhage after tooth extraction in patients undergoing continuous infusion with unfractionated heparin. J Oral Maxillofac Surg. 2012;70(3):521–6.

Vitamin K Antagonists

21

Branislav V. Bajkin and Ivana Urosevic

21.1 Mechanism of Action, Pharmacokinetics and Pharmacodynamics of Vitamin K Antagonists

Oral anticoagulants are pharmacologic agents that reduce the levels of vitamin K-dependent coagulation factors by inhibiting their synthesis. For this reason, these drugs are referred to as vitamin K antagonists (VKAs). The most commonly used agents in this group are the coumarin-derived anticoagulants: acenocoumarol, warfarin, and phenprocoumon. The clinical use of indandione derivatives has been largely abandoned because of the high incidence of allergic reactions.

Coumarin derivatives act by inhibiting the cyclic interconversion of vitamin K and its 2,3-epoxide. Vitamin K, as a cofactor, is required for the carboxylation of glutamate to γ-carboxyglutamate at the N-terminal region of vitamin K-dependent coagulation factors (FII, FVII, FIX, and FX) and anticoagulant proteins C, S, and Z (Fig. 21.1). γ-Carboxylation of vitamin K-dependent proteins is necessary for their biological activity. By blocking the enzyme vitamin K epoxide reductase, VKAs prevent the conversion of vitamin K epoxide to the active reduced form of vitamin K, leading to the hepatic synthesis of partially decarboxylated proteins with reduced activity [1–4].

Coumarin derivatives antagonize vitamin K through a competitive mechanism. Competition is enabled by the presence of similar chemical groups in vitamin K and these drugs. Therapeutic administration or increased dietary intake of vitamin K can diminish the efficacy of VKAs. Patients treated with high doses of vitamin K may develop resistance to coumarin derivatives for up to a week due to hepatic storage

B. V. Bajkin (✉)
University of Novi Sad, Faculty of Medicine, Dentistry Clinic of Vojvodina, Novi Sad, Serbia
e-mail: branislav.bajkin@mf.uns.ac.rs

I. Urosevic
University of Novi Sad, Faculty of Medicine, University Clinical Center of Vojvodina, Clinic of Hematology, Novi Sad, Serbia

B. V. Bajkin (ed.), *Bleeding Disorders and Dentistry*,
https://doi.org/10.1007/978-3-032-26713-9_21

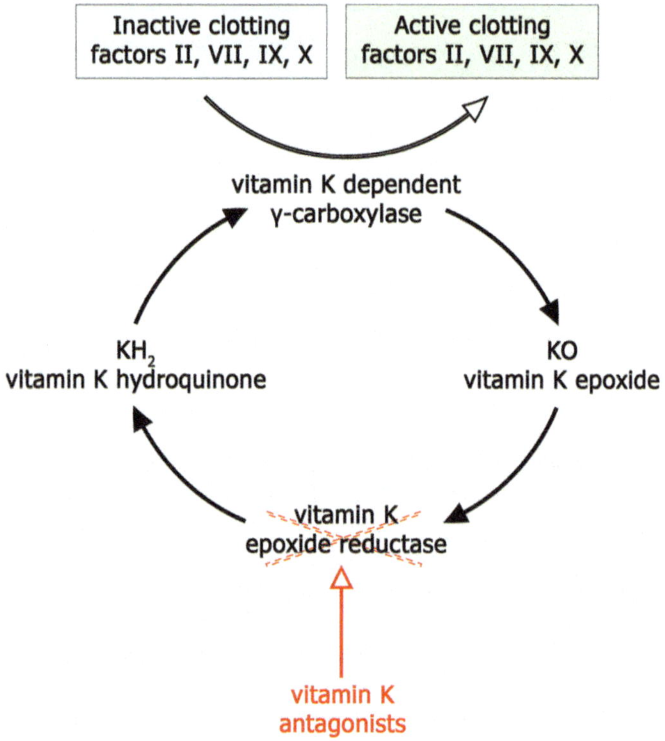

Fig. 21.1 Mechanism of action of vitamin K antagonists

of vitamin K. VKAs are rapidly absorbed from the gastrointestinal tract, highly bound to plasma proteins, metabolized in the liver by hydroxylation, and excreted in urine. These agents have different half-lives, ranging from 8–10 h for acenocoumarol and 36–42 h for warfarin to approximately 150 h for phenprocoumon [1–4].

In contrast to heparin, which exerts an almost immediate effect, VKAs have a delayed onset of action because it takes time for the already synthesized coagulation factors to be cleared from the circulation. The onset of action of VKAs is gradual and depends on the half-lives of the coagulation factors, which are as follows: FVII 4–6 h, FIX and FX 18–24 h, and FII 72 h. The therapeutic anticoagulant effect is typically achieved 2–7 days after treatment initiation. For warfarin, this period usually lasts 4–5 days. When a rapid anticoagulant effect is required, therapy is initiated with unfractionated heparin (UFH) or low molecular weight heparins (LMWHs), while VKAs are introduced concurrently. Once the therapeutic effect of VKAs is established, heparin is withdrawn. Following discontinuation of VKAs, their effect persists for several days, due to the time required for complete drug elimination and the synthesis of new, active vitamin K-dependent coagulation factors [1–3].

The patient's response to VKAs therapy is highly individual and depends on various factors such as diet, the intake and absorption of vitamin K in particular, genetic variations affecting drug metabolism (e.g., cytochrome P450 enzyme CYP2C9 polymorphisms), variations in the vitamin K epoxide reductase enzyme, the presence of comorbidities, age, and interactions with other drugs [3, 4].

21.2 Indications for the Use and Monitoring of Oral Anticoagulant Therapy

Indications for VKA therapy include numerous diseases and conditions, such as primary prevention of venous thrombosis, treatment of deep vein thrombosis (DVT) and/or pulmonary thromboembolism (PE), prevention of recurrent thromboembolism, heart valve replacement and heart valve diseases, atrial fibrillation, before and after cardioversion, dilated cardiomyopathy, and some rare diseases, including antiphospholipid syndrome, congenital thrombophilia, and paroxysmal nocturnal hemoglobinuria. In patients with ischemic coronary and cerebrovascular disease without associated atrial fibrillation, antiplatelet therapy is typically used. Combined antiplatelet and anticoagulant therapy may also be considered, especially in patients at high risk of venous and arterial thromboembolic events [2, 5–12].

Because of their narrow therapeutic range, VKAs require regular monitoring to ensure therapeutic efficacy and safety. The therapeutic effect of these agents is monitored by measuring prothrombin time (PT), which is influenced by the concentrations of three of the four vitamin K-dependent coagulation factors (FII, FVII, and FX). According to the World Health Organization's 1983 recommendation, PT is expressed as the International Normalized Ratio (INR), calculated as follows:

$$\text{INR} = \left(\text{patient's PT} / \text{mean normal PT}\right)^{\text{ISI}},$$

where ISI (International Sensitivity Index) is the sensitivity of thromboplastin used as a reagent for PT measurement.

The therapeutic INR range is the interval of INR values at which the risk of thromboembolism is maximally reduced with minimal risk of bleeding. According to recommendations from the American College of Chest Physicians and the American Heart Association, the therapeutic INR range is 2.0–3.0, except in high-risk patients (e.g., those with mechanical heart valves), for whom a higher range of 2.5–3.5 is advised (Table 21.1) [1, 2, 4]. The European Society of Cardiology and

Table 21.1 Therapeutic INR range in patients taking VKAs

Indications for VKAs	INR range
Deep vein thrombosis prophylaxis	2.0–3.0
Deep vein thrombosis treatment	2.0–3.0
Pulmonary embolism treatment	2.0–3.0
Atrial fibrillation and systemic embolism prevention	2.0–3.0
Mechanical heart valves	2.5–3.5

INR-International Normalized Ratio, *VKAs* vitamin K antagonists the British Committee for Standards in Haematology provided similar recommendations, but in patients with prosthetic heart valves and additional risk factors, slightly higher INR values are suggested (target INR, 3.5; range, 3.0–4.0) [8, 13].

21.3 Interaction of VKAs with Drugs Used in Dental Practice

Many drugs can increase or decrease the effect of VKAs, and when they are used, it is necessary to monitor the INR more frequently and adjust the dose of coumarin derivatives. The effect of VKAs depends, among other things, on the degree of binding to plasma proteins and the rate of metabolism. Many drugs enhance the anticoagulant effect of VKAs by displacing them from plasma protein binding sites, thereby increasing the active, unbound fraction of the drug. The majority of drug interactions affecting warfarin involve inhibition of the CYP2C9 enzyme, which can increase the risk of serious bleeding in patients taking warfarin. On the other hand, the use of medications that induce CYP2C9 results in increased liver metabolism of warfarin and thus less anticoagulation [14].

The most commonly used drugs in dental practice that may affect the action of VKAs include carbamazepine, metronidazole, erythromycin, sulfonamides, tetracyclines, and miconazole (oral gel) (Table 21.2). With the exception of carbamazepine, which accelerates VKA metabolism, all other agents increase the effect of coumarin derivatives [1, 15–19]. Certain herbal preparations, such as St. John's wort, may also affect the effect of coumarin derivatives by reducing their anticoagulant effect.

Antibiotics and Antifungal Agents

Prolonged oral administration of any broad-spectrum antibiotic can suppress the normal gastrointestinal bacterial flora, reducing endogenous vitamin K production and potentiating the effect of VKAs. Drugs such as metronidazole, erythromycin, ciprofloxacin, cotrimoxazole, fluconazole, itraconazole, ketoconazole, miconazole, ofloxacin, aztreonam, chloramphenicol, and sulfonamides should be avoided because of their unpredictable

Table 21.2 Interactions of VKAs and drugs used in dentistry

Drug group	Drug	Effect on VKAs
Analgesics	Aspirin and other NSAIDs Tramadol	Increased
Antibacterials	Metronidazole, erythromycin, cephalosporins, ciprofloksacin, co-trimoxazole, sulfonamides, tetracycline, ampicillin, amoxicillin*	Increased
Antifungals	Ketoconazole, fluconazole, itraconazole, miconazole (oral gel)	Increased
Anticonvulsants	Carbamazepine	Decreased

VKAs vitamin K antagonists, *NSAIDs* nonsteroidal anti-inflammatory drugs

*Prolonged oral antibiotic use may enhance the effect of VKAs due to gut flora suppression, but single dose of amoxicillin used for antibiotic prophylaxis against infective endocarditis does not interfere with the effect of VKAs

effects on VKAs. These drugs may potentiate the anticoagulant activity of coumarin derivatives and cause bleeding complications [3]. In cases requiring prolonged antibiotic therapy, clindamycin is considered the antibiotic of choice for these patients. A single prophylactic dose of antibiotics administered for the prevention of infective endocarditis is considered not to affect the efficacy of coumarin derivatives and does not lead to an increase in INR values [20].

Analgesics

In patients undergoing VKA therapy, the use of acetylsalicylic acid and other non-steroidal anti-inflammatory drugs (NSAIDs) should be avoided. These drugs, in addition to their antiplatelet effect, can cause severe gastrointestinal bleeding by irritating the gastric mucosa. Acetaminophen is considered the analgesic of choice in patients on VKA therapy. Only at higher doses, above 1.5 g per day, and with prolonged use can it potentiate the effects of coumarin derivatives [3, 17, 18]. There are some controversies in the literature regarding the use of selective COX-2 inhibitors (COX-2 inhibitors). It is generally stated that the use of COX-2 inhibitors may be considered safe. However, some studies suggest that these drugs may also cause upper gastrointestinal bleeding [21]. Furthermore, COX-2 inhibitors may lead to an increase in INR values [20].

21.4 Complications of Vitamin K Antagonist Therapy

The most common and most severe complication of VKA treatment is bleeding. Bleeding may occur spontaneously, due to trauma, or secondary to an invasive medical procedure. It can be mild, presenting as ecchymoses, epistaxis, or subconjunctival hemorrhage, or more severe, including extensive hematomas, intracranial hemorrhage, as well as gastrointestinal and genitourinary bleeding. The risk of spontaneous bleeding is associated with the intensity of the anticoagulant effect of VKAs and increases with rising INR. The risk is particularly pronounced when the INR exceeds the recommended therapeutic range.

Treatment of an elevated INR includes temporarily discontinuing anticoagulant therapy or administering vitamin K (orally or intravenously). In cases of severe bleeding, treatment includes infusing fresh frozen plasma (FFP), activated prothrombin complex concentrate (aPCC), or recombinant activated factor VII (rFVIIa). The therapeutic approach depends on the INR level and the severity of bleeding [1, 2, 4].

VKAs have the potential to induce skin necrosis. These drugs may reduce bone density by inhibiting the synthesis of bone proteins, a fact of clinical relevance for dentists. The extent to which the jawbones may be affected by this process has not been sufficiently researched.

References

1. Ansell J, Hirsh J, Hylek E, Jacobson A, Crowther M, Palareti G, American College of Chest Physicians. Pharmacology and management of the vitamin K antagonists: American College of Chest Physicians Evidence-Based Clinical Practice Guidelines (8th edition). Chest. 2008;133(6 Suppl):160S–98S.
2. Hirsh J, Fuster V, Ansell J, Halperin JL. American Heart Association/American College of Cardiology Foundation guide to warfarin therapy. Circulation. 2003;107(12):1692–711.
3. Baglin T. Drugs and haemostasis. In: Bennet PN, Brown MJ, Sharma P, editors. Clinical pharmacology. 11th ed. Churchill Livingstone: Elsevier; 2012. p. 482–95.
4. Weitz JI. Antiplatelet, anticoagulant, and fibrinolytic drugs. In section: Disorders of hemostasis. In: Harrison's principles of internal medicine. 20th ed. McGraw-Hill Education eBook; 2018. p. 843–58.
5. Albers GW, Amarenco P, Easton JD, Sacco RL, Teal P, American College of Chest Physicians. Antithrombotic and thrombolytic therapy for ischemic stroke: American College of Chest Physicians Evidence-Based Clinical Practice Guidelines (8th edition). Chest. 2008;133(6 Suppl):630S–69S.
6. Butchart EG, Gohlke-Bärwolf C, Antunes MJ, Tornos P, De Caterina R, Cormier B, et al. Working Groups on Valvular Heart Disease, Thrombosis, and Cardiac Rehabilitation and Exercise Physiology, European Society of Cardiology. Recommendations for the management of patients after heart valve surgery. Eur Heart J. 2005;26(22):2463–71.
7. Kearon C, Kahn SR, Agnelli G, Goldhaber S, Raskob GE, Comerota AJ, American College of Chest Physicians. Antithrombotic therapy for venous thromboembolic disease: American College of Chest Physicians Evidence-Based Clinical Practice Guidelines (8th edition). Chest. 2008;133(6 Suppl):454S–545S.
8. Keeling D, Baglin T, Tait C, Watson H, Perry D, Baglin C, British Committee for Standards in Haematology, et al. Guidelines on oral anticoagulation with warfarin-fourth edition. Br J Haematol. 2011;154:311–24.
9. Levy S, Breithardt G, Campbell RW, Camm AJ, Daubert JC, Allessie M, et al. Atrial fibrillation: current knowledge and recommendations for management. Working Group on Arrhythmias of the European Society of Cardiology. Eur Heart J. 1998;19(9):1294–320.
10. Lung B, Gohlke-Bärwolf C, Tornos P, Tribouilloy C, Hall R, Butchart E, Vahanian A, Working Group on Valvular Heart Disease. Recommendations on the management of the asymptomatic patient with valvular heart disease. Eur Heart J. 2002;23(16):1252–66.
11. Salem DN, O'Gara PT, Madias C, Pauker SG, American College of Chest Physicians. Valvular and structural heart disease: American College of Chest Physicians Evidence-Based Clinical Practice Guidelines (8th edition). Chest. 2008;133(6 Suppl):593S–629S.
12. Singer DE, Albers GW, Dalen JE, Fang MC, Go AS, Halperin JL, Lip GY, Manning WJ, American College of Chest Physicians. Antithrombotic therapy in atrial fibrillation: American College of Chest Physicians Evidence-Based Clinical Practice Guidelines (8h ed). Chest. 2008;133(6 Suppl):546S–92S.
13. Gohlke-Bärwolf C, Acar J, Oakley C, Butchart E, Burckhardt D, Bodnar E, et al. Guidelines for prevention of thromboembolic events in valvular heart disease. Study group of the working group on valvular heart disease of the European Society of Cardiology. Eur Heart J. 1995;16(10):1320–30.
14. Mar PL, Gopinathannair R, Gengler BE, Chung MK, Perez A, Dukes J, Ezekowitz MD, Lakkireddy D, Lip GYH, Miletello M, Noseworthy PA, Reiffel J, Tisdale JE, Olshansky B, From the American Heart Association Electrocardiography & Arrhythmias Committee of the Council of Clinical Cardiology. Drug interactions affecting oral anticoagulant use. Circ Arrhythm Electrophysiol. 2022;15(6):e007956.
15. Carter G, Goss AN, Lloyd J, Tocchetti R. Current concepts of the management of dental extractions for patients taking warfarin. Aust Dent J. 2003;48(2):89–96.

16. du Breuil AL, Umland EM. Outpatient management of anticoagulation therapy. Am Fam Physician. 2007;75(7):1031–42.
17. Scully C, Wolff A. Oral surgery in patients on anticoagulant therapy. Oral Surg Oral Med Oral Pathol Oral Radiol Endod. 2002;94:57–64.
18. Scully C. Haemathology. In: Scully's medical problems in dentistry. 7th ed. Churchill Livingstone: Elsevier; 2014. p. 212–75.
19. Little JW, Miller CS, Rhodus NL. Acquired bleeding and hypercoagulable disorders. In: Little and Falace's dental management of the medically compromised patient. 9th ed. St. Louis: Elsevier; 2018. p. 428–56.
20. Perry DJ, Noakes TJC, Helliwell PS. Guidelines for the management of patients on oral anticoagulants requiring dental surgery. Br Dent J. 2007;203:389–93.
21. Villa Zapata L, Hansten PD, Panic J, Horn JR, Boyce RD, Gephart S, Subbian V, Romero A, Malone DC. Risk of bleeding with exposure to warfarin and nonsteroidal anti-inflammatory drugs: a systematic review and meta-analysis. Thromb Haemost. 2020;120(7):1066–74.

Dental Management in Patients Taking Vitamin K Antagonists

22

Branislav V. Bajkin and Alison Dougall

Box 22.1 Dental Management of Patients Taking Vitamin K Antagonists

Coumarin derivatives

Acenocoumarol
Warfarin
Phenprocoumon

Oral surgery in patients taking VKA

- Consult the patient's physician to discuss the risk of bleeding and the risk of thromboembolism
- INR should be checked on the day of the procedure. In a patient with stable INR values, checking the INR no more than 48–72 h before the procedure is acceptable
- If INR is within the therapeutic range (<4.0)*, dental extractions, simple implant placement and other minor oral surgical procedures are considered to be safe without discontinuing VKA
- If INR is >4.0, invasive dental treatment should be delayed until reduction of INR
- In a case of more extensive surgery (full mouth extraction, difficult third molar surgery, periodontal surgery, soft and bone tissue augmentation procedures, orthognathic surgery etc.) temporary cessation of VKA with or without LMWH bridging therapy should be considered in consultation

(continued)

B. V. Bajkin (✉)
University of Novi Sad, Faculty of Medicine, Dentistry Clinic of Vojvodina, Novi Sad, Serbia
e-mail: branislav.bajkin@mf.uns.ac.rs

A. Dougall
School of Dental Science, Trinity College Dublin, Dublin Dental University Hospital, Dublin, Ireland

B. V. Bajkin (ed.), *Bleeding Disorders and Dentistry*,
https://doi.org/10.1007/978-3-032-26713-9_22

Box 22.1 (continued)

with patient's physician. The risk of thromboembolism has to be estimated. Modification of anticoagulant treatment should be initiated and carefully planned by patient's physicians

- Avoid prolonged antibiotic use and the use of other drugs that may interfere with VKA effect
- Schedule a patient at the beginning of the work week
- IANB is considered to be safe in therapeutically anticoagulated patients
- Use of local anesthesia with adrenalin, if not otherwise contraindicated
- Minimally traumatic surgical technique; multiple appointments may be necessary; consider carrying out the treatments in a stage manner, if possible
- Use of local hemostatic agents and measures to control oral bleeding; suturing of postextraction socket should be considered
- For pain relief use acetaminophen if not contraindicated; avoid aspirin and NSAIDs
- Provide a patient with postoperative instructions (soft and cold diet, phone number in case of an emergency) and regular follow-up
- In a patient receiving combined VKA and antiplatelet therapy there is a higher risk of postoperative bleeding but there is no need for cessation of either VKA or antiplatelet therapy for simple tooth extractions and other minor oral surgical procedures, if INR is within therapeutic range and local hemostasis measures are used

VKA vitamin K antagonists, *INR* International Normalized Ratio, *IANB* inferior alveolar nerve block, *NSAIDs* nonsteroidal anti-inflammatory drugs

*According to some authors and recommendations INR should not exceed 3.5

22.1 Local Anesthesia and Pain Management in Patients Taking Vitamin K Antagonists

In addition to bleeding from surgical wounds, patients receiving vitamin K antagonists (VKAs) are at risk of hematoma formation as a complication of local anesthesia. The risk of hemorrhage associated with the inferior alveolar nerve block (IANB) is the greatest concern. Minor bleeding within the pterygomandibular space can cause trismus, whereas more severe hemorrhage can result in airway obstruction. In contrast to any technique of block anesthesia in persons with hemophilia, particularly IANB, which requires factor replacement therapy, this local anesthesia technique is not considered excessively risky in patients receiving VKAs, provided their INR is within the therapeutic range [1–3]. For IANB, it is recommended to use carpule syringes and thinner needles (27 G), perform mandatory aspiration, apply local anesthetics slowly (1 mL over 60 s), and use a local anesthetic containing a vasoconstrictor. However, whenever possible, preference should always be given to safer local anesthesia techniques, such as local infiltration or intraligamentary anesthesia.

Paracetamol is considered the analgesic of choice when not contraindicated. NSAIDs such as aspirin, ibuprofen, diclofenac, and naproxen should be avoided because of their antiplatelet effect and the irritation of the gastric mucosa, which can cause severe gastrointestinal bleeding.

22.2 Oral Surgery in Patients Taking Vitamin K Antagonists

Given the frequency of tooth extractions in dental practice, it is not surprising that the majority of research has focused on dental extractions in patients receiving VKAs and that most practical recommendations in the literature have been derived from studies assessing the risk of bleeding following this oral surgical procedure. In the past, dose reduction or temporary discontinuation of VKA therapy, with or without heparin bridging, was commonly advocated before a tooth extraction. It is important to emphasize that such an approach exposes the patient to a risk of thromboembolism, which varies among patients (see Chap. 18). It also has to be acknowledged that replacing one anticoagulant with another during bridging therapy does not entirely eliminate the risk of hemorrhage. Therefore, such an approach for simple tooth extraction is not recommended [4, 5].

Results from numerous studies and systematic literature reviews indicate that tooth extractions and other dentoalveolar surgical procedures can be safely performed without interrupting oral anticoagulant therapy, provided the INR is within the therapeutic range, a minimally traumatic surgical technique is used, and appropriate local hemostatic measures are applied [6–9]. Similar recommendations have been issued by numerous professional associations [2, 10–13].

Recent literature reports very few cases of postextraction bleeding in patients receiving VKA therapy that could not be managed with local hemostatic measures [4]. The use of minimally traumatic surgical techniques and local hemostatic measures are of great importance in oral surgery. Risk factors for postoperative bleeding include high INR, local inflammation, extent of oral surgery, and the concomitant use of antiplatelet and anticoagulant therapy [14].

The upper limit of the therapeutic INR range is 3.5 or 4.0, and these values should be considered the maximum acceptable threshold for tooth extraction (Fig. 22.1a, b). When INR is within the therapeutic range, the incidence of postextraction bleeding is expected to be higher in patients with higher INR values. However, contradictory data are reported in the literature, ranging from studies that confirm this assumption [15, 16] to those that do not report such an association [17–21].

Local inflammation should be considered a risk factor for postoperative bleeding. In patients on VKA therapy undergoing multiple tooth extractions, prolonged bleeding, if it occurs, is usually not observed at all extraction sites but rather at those with pronounced local inflammation [5].

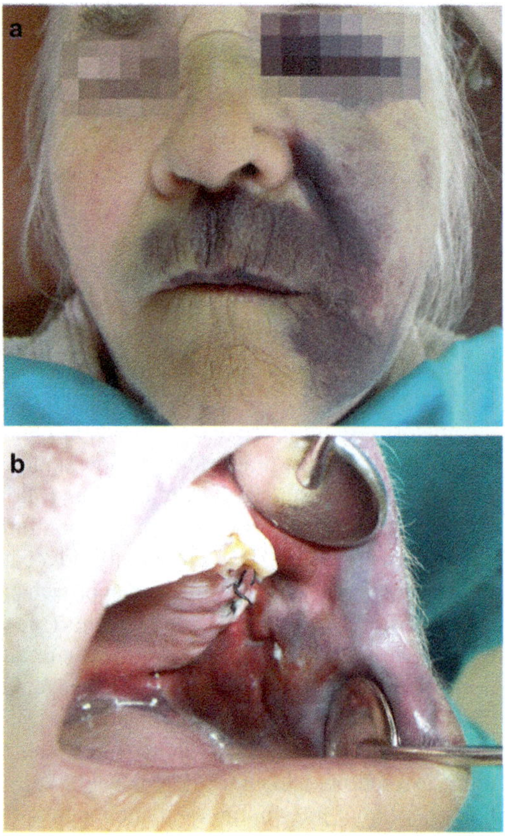

Fig. 22.1 (**a**) Facial hematoma after tooth extraction in a patient overdosed with vitamin K antagonists (INR > 8). (**b**) Intraoral hematoma in the patient shown in (**a**), spreading through the soft tissues with a risk of airway obstruction

The literature emphasizes the importance of minimally traumatic surgical techniques during oral surgery in patients receiving oral anticoagulant therapy. The degree of surgical trauma influences the risk of postoperative bleeding. Extraction of up to three teeth is considered safe in patients with INR values within the therapeutic range [2, 22, 23]. For more extensive oral surgical procedures, such as multiple extractions, third molar surgery, and other procedures requiring raising of a mucoperiosteal flap, the decision should be based on a risk assessment of bleeding versus the risk of thromboembolism if therapy is interrupted. Studies indicate that effective local hemostasis can be achieved even after more extensive dentoalveolar surgical procedures [14]. For more extensive procedures in the head or neck region, temporary discontinuation of VKAs with heparin bridging is the treatment of choice in most cases.

For the prevention and management of postoperative bleeding following dentoalveolar surgical procedures in patients on VKA therapy, various local hemostatic agents may be used, including oxidized regenerated cellulose [18, 20, 24–26], absorbable gelatin sponge [17, 18, 20], absorbable collagen products [5, 14, 19], fibrin glue, cyanoacrylate adhesive [27], platelet-rich plasma [28], and antifibrinolytics in the form of a mouthwash solution [24, 29], along with suturing of the extraction site. Studies comparing the efficacy of different local hemostatic agents have not shown a clear advantage of any specific product [17, 30, 31].

22.3 Implant Surgery in Patients Taking Vitamin K Antagonists

The surgical trauma associated with implant placement is similar to that during tooth extraction [32, 33]. However, some suggest that dental implant surgery should be considered a high-risk procedure in patients undergoing VKA therapy [2, 34]. Severe bleeding following implant placement has been reported in the literature, even in patients without bleeding disorders. Bleeding may occur following a sinus lift [35, 36] and in the floor of the mouth, usually as a result of perforation of the lingual cortical bone and injury to the sublingual blood vessels during implant site preparation [37, 38]. It is reasonable to assume that anticoagulant therapy could further exacerbate such conditions, so dental implant surgery in these patients requires additional caution.

A limited number of studies addressing dental implant procedures in patients undergoing VKA therapy are available in the literature [22, 39–42]. Most authors advocate no need to temporarily interrupt VKAs for dental implant placement, provided the INR is within the therapeutic range [43–46]. However, dental implant surgery often requires more extensive procedures, such as bone augmentation, sinus lift, and bone and soft tissue grafts. These procedures require careful planning, and the decision to continue or interrupt therapy should be made in consultation with the physician, based on an assessment of the bleeding risk versus the risk of thrombosis if therapy is discontinued [43, 44]. Given the increasing trend in dental implant procedures, it is very likely that future research involving patients on anticoagulant therapy will focus more on dental implantology than on tooth extractions.

22.4 Oral Surgery in Patients on Combined Oral Anticoagulant and Antiplatelet Therapy

In patients at high risk of thromboembolic complications, particularly those with a concurrent risk of both arterial and venous thrombosis, a combined therapeutic approach with VKAs and antiplatelet agents may be considered. Combined anticoagulant/antiplatelet treatment is indicated in patients receiving VKAs who also require cardiovascular prophylaxis. Aspirin is the most commonly used antiplatelet agent and is usually administered at prophylactic doses not exceeding 100 mg.

Despite the benefits of combined therapy, these patients are at increased risk of spontaneous bleeding or bleeding after trauma or surgery [47–49]. On the other hand, discontinuing either VKAs or antiplatelet therapy for surgical intervention increases the risk of thromboembolism [50, 51].

During dental treatment in these patients, the increased risk of bleeding should be considered, and surgical procedures should be discussed with the patient's physician. Research findings suggest that minor oral surgical procedures, including tooth extractions, can be safely performed in patients on combined VKAs and antiplatelet therapy without interrupting treatment, provided the INR is within the therapeutic range [21, 52, 53]. Modification of the therapeutic regimen should be considered in cases of extensive surgery.

In addition to assessing the risk of bleeding versus the risk of thromboembolism, comorbidities that may further complicate the dental procedure should be considered when treatment is modified. For elective surgical procedures, the procedure may be temporarily postponed, particularly following recent thromboembolic events, until the patient's general health is stabilized.

References

1. Bajkin BV, Todorovic LM. Safety of local anaesthesia in dental patients taking oral anticoagulants: is it still controversial? Br J Oral Maxillofac Surg. 2012;50:65–8.
2. Scottish Dental Clinical Effectiveness Programme. Management of dental patients taking anticoagulants or antiplatelet drugs. Dental clinical guidance. 2nd ed; 2022. Available online at: https://www.sdcep.org.uk/media/ypnl2cpz/sdcep-management-of-dental-patients-taking-anticoagulants-or-antiplatelet-drugs-2nd-edition.pdf. Accessed June 2024.
3. Wahl MJ, Miller CS, Rhodus NL, Kämmerer P, Dinkova A, Lalla RV, Bajkin BV. Anticoagulants are dental friendly. Oral Surg Oral Med Oral Pathol Oral Radiol. 2018;125(2):103–6.
4. Wahl MJ. Perioperative management of dental patients on anticoagulants. In: Szumita RP, Szumita PM, editors. Hemostasis in dentistry. Cham: Springer; 2018. p. 151–86.
5. Bajkin BV, Popovic SL, Selakovic SDJ. Randomized, prospective trial comparing bridging therapy using low-molecular-weight heparin with maintenance of oral anticoagulation during extraction of teeth. J Oral Maxillofac Surg. 2009;67(5):990–5.
6. Kämmerer PW, Frerich B, Liese J, Schiegnitz E, Al-Nawas B. Oral surgery during therapy with anticoagulants-a systematic review. Clin Oral Investig. 2015;19:171–80.
7. Kosyfaki P, Att W, Strub JR. The dental patient on oral anticoagulant medication: a literature review. J Oral Rehabil. 2011;38:615–33.
8. Nematullah A, Alabousi A, Blanas N, Douketis JD, Sutherland SE. Dental surgery for patients on anticoagulant therapy with warfarin: a systematic review and meta-analysis. J Can Dent Assoc. 2009;75(1):41–41i.
9. Shi Q, Xu J, Zhang T, Zhang B, Liu H. Post-operative bleeding risk in dental surgery for patients on oral anticoagulant therapy: a meta-analysis of observational studies. Front Pharmacol. 2017;8:58.
10. American Dental Association. Oral anticoagulant and antiplatelet medications and dental procedures. Available online at: https://www.ada.org/resources/research/science-and-research-institute/oral-health-topics/oral-anticoagulant-and-antiplatelet-medications-and-dental-procedures. Accessed June 2024.
11. Armstrong MJ, Gronseth G, Anderson DC, Biller J, Cucchiara B, Dafer R, Goldstein LB, Schneck M, Messé SR. Summary of evidence-based guideline: periprocedural management of antithrombotic medications in patients with ischemic cerebrovascular disease. Report of the Guideline Development Subcommittee of the American Academy of Neurology. Neurology. 2013;80(22):2065–9.

12. Douketis JD, Spyropoulos AC, Spencer FA, Mayr M, Jaffer AK, Eckman MH, et al. Perioperative management of antithrombotic therapy. Antithrombotic therapy and prevention of thrombosis, 9th ed.: American College of Chest Physicians Evidence-Based Clinical Practice Guidelines. Chest. 2012;141(2 Suppl):e326–e350S.
13. Durso SC. Oral manifestations of disease. In section: Disorders of eyes, ears, nose and throat. In: Harrison's principles of internal medicine. 20th ed. McGraw-Hill Education eBook; 2018. p. 219–25.
14. Bajkin BV, Vujkov SB, Milekic BR, Vuckovic BA. Risk factors for bleeding after oral surgery in patients who continued using oral anticoagulant therapy. J Am Dent Assoc. 2015;146(6):375–81.
15. Al-Mubarak S, Al-Ali N, Abou-Rass M, Al-Sohail A, Robert A, Al-Zoman K, et al. Evaluation of dental extractions, suturing and INR on postoperative bleeding of patients maintained on oral anticoagulant therapy. Br Dent J. 2007;203(7):e15.
16. Al- Mubarak S, Rass MA, Alsuwyed A, Alabdulaaly A, Ciancio S. Thromboembolic risk and bleeding in patients maintaining or stopping oral anticoagulant therapy during dental extraction. J Throm Haemost. 2006;4:89–91.
17. Blinder D, Manor Y, Martinovitz U, Taicher S. Dental extractions in patients maintained on oral anticoagulant therapy: comparison of INR value with occurrence of postoperative bleeding. Int J Oral Maxillofac Surg. 2001;30:518–21.
18. Salam S, Yusuf H, Milosevic A. Bleeding after dental extractions in patients taking warfarin. Br J Oral Maxillofac Surg. 2007;45:463–6.
19. Bodner L, Weinstein JM, Baumgarten AK. Efficacy of fibrin sealant in patients on various levels of oral anticoagulant undergoing oral surgery. Oral Surg Oral Med Oral Pathol Oral Radiol Endod. 1998;86(4):421–4.
20. Zanon E, Martinelli F, Bacci C, Cordioli G, Girolami A. Safety of dental extraction among consecutive patients on oral anticoagulant treatment managed using a specific dental management protocol. Blood Coagul Fibrinolisis. 2003;14(1):27–30.
21. Morimoto Y, Niwa H, Minematsu K. Hemostatic management of tooth extractions in patients on oral antithrombotic therapy. J Oral Maxillofac Surg. 2008;66:51–7.
22. Broekema FI, Minnen B, Jansma J, Bos RR. Risk of bleeding after dentoalveolar surgery in patients taking anticoagulants. Br J Oral Maxillofac Surg. 2014;52(3):e15–9.
23. Scully C. Haemathology. In: Scully's medical problems in dentistry. 7th ed. Elsevier: Churchill Livingstone; 2014. p. 212–75.
24. Carter G, Goss A. Tranexamic acid mouthwash-a prospective randomized study of a 2-day regimen vs 5-day regimen to prevent postoperative bleeding in anticoagulated patients requiring dental extractions. Int J Oral Maxillofac Surg. 2003;32(5):504–7.
25. Devani P, Lavery KM, Howell CJT. Dental extractions in patients on warfarin: is alteration of anticoagulant regime necessary? Br J Oral Maxillofac Surg. 1998;36:107–11.
26. Sacco R, Sacco M, Carpenedo M, Mannucci PM. Oral surgery in patients on oral anticoagulant therapy: a randomized comparison of different intensity targets. Oral Surg Oral Med Oral Pathol Oral Radiol Endod. 2007;104:e18–21.
27. Al-Belasy FA, Amer MZ. Hemostatic effect of n-butyl-2-cyanoacrylate (histoacryl) glue in warfarin-treated patients undergoing oral surgery. J Oral Maxillofac Surg. 2003;61(12):1405–9.
28. Della Valle A, Sammartino G, Marenzi G, Tia M, Espedito di Lauro A, Ferrari F, et al. Prevention of postoperative bleeding in anticoagulated patients undergoing oral surgery: use of platelet rich plasma gel. J Oral Maxillofac Surg. 2003;61(11):1275–8.
29. Sindet-Pedersen S, Ramstrom G, Bernvil S, Blomback M. Hemostatic effect of tranexamic acid mouthwash in anticoagulant-treated patients undergoing oral surgery. N Engl J Med. 1989;320(13):840–3.
30. Carter G, Goss A, Lloyd J, Tocchetti R. Tranexamic acid mouthwash versus autologous fibrin glue in patients taking warfarin undergoing dental extractions: a randomized prospective clinical study. J Oral Maxillofac Surg. 2003;61(12):1432–5.

31. Halfpenny W, Fraser JS, Adlam DM. Comparison of 2 hemostatic agents for the prevention of postextraction hemorrhage in patients on anticoagulants. Oral Surg Oral Med Oral Pathol Oral Radiol Endod. 2001;92(3):257–9.
32. Madrid C, Sanz M. What influence do anticoagulants have on oral implant therapy? A systematic review. Clin Oral Implants Res. 2009;20(Suppl 4):96–106.
33. Sanz M, Naert I. Biomechanics/risk management (Working Group 2). Clin Oral Implants Res. 2009;20(Suppl 4):107–11.
34. Zeevi I, Allon DM, Rosenfeld E, Avishai G, Gilman L, Nissan J, Chaushu G. Four-year cross-sectional study of bleeding risk in dental patients on direct anticoagulants. Quintessence Int. 2017;48(6):503–9.
35. Jensen SS, Eriksen J, Schiødt M. Severe bleeding after sinus floor elevation using the transcrestal technique: a case report. Eur J Oral Implantol. 2012;5(3):287–91.
36. Hong YH, Mun SK. A case of massive maxillary sinus bleeding after dental implant. Int J Oral Maxillofac Surg. 2011;40(7):758–60.
37. Kalpidis CDR, Setayesh RM. Hemorrhaging associated with endosseus implant placement in the anterior mandible: a review of the literature. J Periodontol. 2004;75(5):631–45.
38. Law C, Alam P, Borumandi F. Floor-of-mouth hematoma following dental implant placement: literature review and case presentation. J Oral Maxillofac Surg. 2017;75:2340–6.
39. Bacci C, Berengo M, Favero L, Zanon E. Safety of dental implant surgery in patients undergoing anticoagulation therapy: a prospective case-control study. Clin Oral Implants Res. 2011;22(2):151–6.
40. Clemm R, Neukam FW, Rusche B, Bauersachs A, Musazada S, Schmitt CM. Management of anticoagulated patients in implant therapy: a clinical comparative study. Clin Oral Implants Res. 2016;27(10):1274–82.
41. Rubino RT, Dawson DR 3rd, Kryscio RJ, Al-Sabbagh M, Miller CS. Postoperative bleeding associated with antiplatelet and anticoagulant drugs: a retrospective study. Oral Surg Oral Med Oral Pathol Oral Radiol. 2019;128(3):243–9.
42. Manor Y, Peleg O, Mijiritsky E, Manor A, Reiter S. A retrospective analysis of dental implantation under anticoagulant treatment. Clin Oral Investig. 2021;25(3):1001–9.
43. Bajkin BV, Wahl MJ, Miller CS. Dental implant surgery and risk of bleeding in patients on antithrombotic medications: a review of the literature. Oral Surg Oral Med Oral Pathol Oral Radiol. 2020;130(5):522–32.
44. Dawoud BES, Kent S, Tabbenor O, George P, Dhanda J. Dental implants and risk of bleeding in patients on oral anticoagulants: a systematic review and meta-analysis. Int J Implant Dent. 2021;7(1):82.
45. Zou L, Hua L. Risk of bleeding with dental implant surgery in patients on anticoagulant or antiplatelet drugs: a systematic review and meta-analysis. Acta Odontol Scand. 2023;81(2):98–104.
46. Miziara LNB, Sendyk WR, Ortega KL, Gallottini M, Sendyk DI, Martins F. Risk of bleeding during implant surgery in patients taking antithrombotics: a systematic review. Semin Thromb Hemost. 2021;47(6):702–8.
47. Dentali F, Douketis JD, Lim W, Crowther M. Combined aspirin-oral anticoagulant therapy compared with oral anticoagulant therapy alone among patients at risk for cardiovascular disease: a metaanalysis of randomized trials. Arch Intern Med. 2007;167(2):117–24.
48. Douketis JD, Arneklev K, Goldhaber SZ, Spandorfer J, Halperin F, Horrow J. Comparison of bleeding in patients with nonvalvular atrial fibrillation treated with ximelagatran or warfarin: assessment of incidence, case-fatality rate, time course and sites of bleeding, and risk factors for bleeding. Arch Intern Med. 2006;166(8):853–9.
49. Hansen ML, Sørensen R, Clausen MT, Fog-Petersen ML, Raunsø J, Gadsbøll N, et al. Risk of bleeding with single, dual, or triple therapy with warfarin, aspirin, and clopidogrel in patients with atrial fibrillation. Arch Intern Med. 2010;170(16):1433–41.
50. Biondi-Zoccai GGL, Lotrionte M, Agostoni P, Abbate A, Fusaro M, Burzotta F, et al. A systematic review and meta-analysis on the hazards of discontinuing or not adhering to aspirin among 50,279 patients at risk for coronary artery disease. Eur Heart J. 2006;27(22):2667–74.

51. Burger W, Chemnitius JM, Kneissl GD, Rücker G. Low-dose aspirin for secondary cardiovascular prevention: cardiovascular risks after its perioperative withdrawal versus bleeding risks with its continuation—review and meta-analysis. J Intern Med. 2005;257(5):399–414.
52. Morimoto Y, Niwa H, Minematsu K. Risk factors affecting postoperative hemorrhage after tooth extraction in patients receiving oral antithrombotic therapy (published online ahead of print Feb. 1, 2011). J Oral Maxillofac Surg. 2011;69(6):1550–6.
53. Bajkin BV, Bajkin IA, Petrovic BB. The effects of combined oral anticoagulant-aspirin therapy in patients undergoing tooth extractions: a prospective study. J Am Dent Assoc. 2012;143(7):771–6.

Direct Oral Anticoagulants

23

Branislav V. Bajkin and Ivana Urosevic

Direct oral anticoagulants (DOACs) were introduced into clinical practice in 2008. Compared with vitamin K antagonists (VKAs), these drugs offer several advantages, including a rapid onset of action (within 1–4 h) through direct inhibition of coagulation factors, a predictable anticoagulant effect without routine monitoring, fixed dosing regimens (once or twice a day), a wider therapeutic window, and significantly fewer food and drug interactions [1–4]. For these reasons, use of these agents has been steadily increasing and is expected to rise in the coming years [5]. DOACs are used to prevent stroke and systemic embolism in patients with non-valvular atrial fibrillation, to prevent and treat deep vein thrombosis and pulmonary thromboembolism, and for thromboprophylaxis in patients undergoing orthopedic hip and knee surgery [1, 6–9]. This group of drugs includes direct thrombin inhibitors and factor Xa (FXa) inhibitors.

Standard laboratory tests, such as prothrombin time (PT, INR) and activated partial thromboplastin time (aPTT) are not reliable for evaluating the anticoagulant effect of DOACs. For the qualitative assessment of the anticoagulant effect of dabigatran, the aPTT can be used, whereas the PT can be used for the qualitative evaluation of the effect of FXa inhibitors, primarily rivaroxaban and edoxaban and to a lesser extent apixaban [1]. More precise tests, such as thrombin clotting time, ecarin clotting time, diluted thrombin time and anti-FXa test, are not routinely used in everyday clinical practice. Even these tests are not reliable enough, as the results depend greatly on the time frame between periods of taking the drug and the moment of testing.

B. V. Bajkin (✉)
University of Novi Sad, Faculty of Medicine, Dentistry Clinic of Vojvodina, Novi Sad, Serbia
e-mail: branislav.bajkin@mf.uns.ac.rs

I. Urosevic
University of Novi Sad, Faculty of Medicine, University Clinical Center of Vojvodina, Clinic of Hematology, Novi Sad, Serbia

B. V. Bajkin (ed.), *Bleeding Disorders and Dentistry*,
https://doi.org/10.1007/978-3-032-26713-9_23

The main adverse effect of DOACs is bleeding. The most severe is intracranial hemorrhage, and the most common is gastrointestinal bleeding. Additionally, there is a risk of prolonged and enhanced bleeding after trauma or surgical interventions. For a mild bleeding event, it is usually sufficient to skip the next one or two doses of the drug. Serious bleeding requires the use of specific antidotes (Table 18.1).

23.1 Direct Thrombin Inhibitors

Dabigatran etexilate (Pradaxa®) is a prodrug whose active form, dabigatran, is poorly absorbed after oral administration. Dabigatran is a direct competitive inhibitor of thrombin. It reversibly inhibits both free and clot-bound thrombin, thereby preventing the conversion of fibrinogen to fibrin. The drug is rapidly absorbed from the gastrointestinal tract and, following plasma hydrolysis, exerts its effect very quickly. It reaches peak plasma concentration within 1.5–4 h. The half-life of the drug is 12–17 h, but in patients with impaired renal function, it may be prolonged to 27 h. Approximately 80%–85% of the drug is not metabolized and is excreted through the kidneys. The drug's dosage and duration of action depend on renal function. It is usually administered at 110 mg or 150 mg, once or twice a day. The effect of the drug lasts for approximately 22 h [2, 3, 10–12].

Idarucizumab, a monoclonal antibody, is a specific antidote for dabigatran and is used in cases of life-threatening bleeding [13, 14]. For mild bleeding events, it is possible to omit a dose or temporarily discontinue dabigatran because of its short half-life.

Routine monitoring of the anticoagulant effect of dabigatran is not recommended. Thrombin and ecarin clotting times are the most sensitive tests, but they are not routinely used in clinical practice. INR (PT) and aPTT are not reliable for assessing the drug's effect [2, 3, 10]. In patients with renal insufficiency, determination of creatinine clearance (CrCl) is recommended. Reduced CrCl (<50 mL/min) indicates slower drug elimination and a potential need to temporarily interrupt dabigatran treatment prior to major surgical interventions.

23.2 Factor Xa Inhibitors

Rivaroxaban (Xarelto®), apixaban (Eliquis®), and edoxaban (Lixiana®, Savaysa®) are FXa inhibitors that prevent the conversion of prothrombin to thrombin. Unlike dabigatran, these drugs are administered in active form. FXa inhibitors have a dual mechanism of action, inhibiting both free and bound FXa, as well as the prothrombinase complex. Rivaroxaban and apixaban inhibit both free and bound FXa and the activity of the prothrombinase complex, whereas edoxaban acts on free FXa and factor FX incorporated into the prothrombinase complex [15, 16]. Studies have shown that these drugs are not inferior to VKAs in preventing stroke and systemic embolism in patients with atrial fibrillation [17, 18].

Rivaroxaban is taken once daily. It is rapidly absorbed from the gastrointestinal tract, reaching peak plasma concentrations within 2.5–4 h. The drug's half-life is 5–9 h, but in elderly patients, it may be prolonged to 12–13 h. Rivaroxaban, like other DOACs, is metabolized in the liver. Cytochrome P450 inhibitors may enhance the effect of rivaroxaban and increase the risk of bleeding. Conversely, cytochrome P450 inducers may reduce the effect of this drug. The anti-Xa assay is considered the most reliable laboratory test for assessing the effect of rivaroxaban. However, as with all DOACs, routine monitoring is not performed [2, 3, 10, 11].

Apixaban is taken orally, twice daily. It reaches peak plasma concentrations approximately 3 h after administration. The drug's half-life is 8–13 h, longer than that of other DOACs. As with rivaroxaban, the anti-Xa assay is considered the most reliable test for assessing the drug's effect, but routine monitoring is not recommended [2, 3, 10, 11]. Andexanet alpha, a recombinant FXa coagulation factor, is a specific antidote for rivaroxaban and apixaban and is used in cases of life-threatening bleeding [14, 19].

Edoxaban is a direct, reversible, and selective FXa inhibitor administered once daily. It reaches peak plasma concentration within 1–2 h after administration, which is faster than with other DOACs. The drug's half-life is 10–14 h. Approximately 50% of the drug is excreted through the kidneys. Although not officially approved, andexanet alfa may serve as an antidote for edoxaban in case of life-threatening bleeding [14].

The pharmacokinetics and clinical implications of DOACs and VKAs relevant to the dental management of patients taking these drugs are shown in Table 23.1.

Table 23.1 Pharmacokinetics and clinical implications of DOACs and VKAs

Drug	Dabigatran	Rivaroxaban	Apixaban	Edoxaban	Warfarin	Acenocoumarol
Target	Thrombin	FXa	FXa	FXa	Vitamin K-dependent factors	Vitamin K-dependent factors
Usual doses and daily administration	150 mg OD or BID	20 mg OD	5 mg BID	60 mg OD	OD, individual dosage	OD, individual dosage
Maximal plasma concentration	1.5–4 h	2.5–4 h	3–4 h	1–2 h	2–6 h	1–3 h
Renal clearance	80%–85%	35%	27%	50%	Less crucial, metabolized by the liver	Less crucial, metabolized by the liver
Half-life	12–17 h	5–9 h	8–13 h	10–14 h	36–42 h	8–11 h
Duration of the effect	Short	Short	Short	Short	Long	Long
Routine laboratory monitoring	No; ECC, TT	No; anti Xa-assay	No; anti Xa-assay	No; anti Xa-assay	INR	INR
Reversal agent	Idaricizumab	Andexanet alfa*			Vitamin K	

VKAs vitamin K antagonists, *DOACs* direct oral anticoagulants, *INR* International Normalized Ratio, *OD* once daily, *BID* twice a day, *FXa* factor Xa, *ECT* ecarin clotting time, *TT* thrombin clotting time

*Andexanet alfa is not officially approved as a reversal agent for edoxaban

References

1. Weitz JI. Antiplatelet, anticoagulant, and fibrinolytic drugs. In section: Disorders of hemostasis. In: Harrison's principles of internal medicine. 20th ed. McGraw-Hill Education eBook; 2018. p. 843–58.
2. Little JW. New oral anticoagulants: will they replace warfarin? Oral Surg Oral Med Oral Pathol Oral Radiol. 2012;113(5):575–80.
3. Firriolo JF, Hupp WS. Beyond warfarin: the new generation of oral anticoagulants and their implications for the management of dental patients. Oral Surg Oral Med Oral Pathol Oral Radiol. 2012;113(4):431–41.
4. Scaglione F. New oral anticoagulants: comparative pharmacology with vitamin K antagonists. Clin Pharmacokinet. 2013;52(2):69–82.
5. Loo SY, Dell'Aniello S, Huiart L, Renoux C. Trends in the prescription of novel oral anticoagulants in UK primary care. Br J Clin Pharmacol. 2017;83(9):2096–106.
6. Connolly S, Ezekowitz M, Yusuf S, Eikelboom J, Oldgren J, Parekh A, et al. Dabigatran versus warfarin in patients with atrial fibrillation. N Engl J Med. 2009;361(12):1139–51.
7. U.S. Food and Drug Administration. FDA approves Pradaxa to prevent stroke in people with atrial fibrillation. FDA News Release; 2010. Available at: https://www.accessdata.fda.gov/drugsatfda_docs/nda/2010/022512Orig1s000Approv.pdf. Accessed June 2024.
8. European Medicines Agency. Available at: https://www.ema.europa.eu/en/documents/product-information/pradaxa-epar-product-information_en.pdf. Accessed June 2024.
9. Chan N, Sobieraj-Teague M, Eikelboom JW. Direct oral anticoagulants: evidence and unresolved issues. Lancet. 2020;396(10264):1767–76.
10. Costantinides F, Rizzo R, Pascazio L, Maglione M. Managing patients taking novel oral anticoagulants (NOAs) in dentistry: a discussion paper on clinical implications. BMC Oral Health. 2016;16:5.
11. Baglin T. Drugs and haemostasis. In: Bennet PN, Brown MJ, Sharma P, editors. Clinical pharmacology. 11th ed. Churchill Livingstone: Elsevier; 2012. p. 482–95.
12. Stangier J, Rathgen K, Stähle H, Gansser D, Roth W. The pharmacokinetics, pharmacodynamics and tolerability of dabigatran etexilate, a new oral direct thrombin inhibitor, in healthy male subjects. Br J Clin Pharmacol. 2007;64(3):292–303.
13. Food and Drug Administration. Praxbind (idarucizumab)—prescribing Information. FDA; 2015. https://www.accessdata.fda.gov/drugsatfda_docs/label/2015/761025lbl.pdf. Accessed June 2024.
14. Scottish Dental Clinical Effectiveness Programme. Management of dental patients taking anticoagulants or antiplatelet drugs. Dental clinical guidance. 2nd ed; 2022. Available online at: https://www.sdcep.org.uk/media/ypnl2cpz/sdcep-management-of-dental-patients-taking-anticoagulants-or-antiplatelet-drugs-2nd-edition.pdf. Accessed June 2024.
15. Gross PL, Weitz JI. New anticoagulants for treatment of venous thromboembolism. Arterioscler Thromb Vasc Biol. 2008;28(3):380–6.
16. Poulakos M, Walker JN, Baig U, David T. Edoxaban: a direct oral anticoagulant. Am J Health Syst Pharm. 2017;74(3):117–29.
17. ROCKET AF Study Investigators. Rivaroxaban-once daily, oral, direct factor Xa inhibition compared with vitamin K antagonism for prevention of stroke and Embolism Trial in Atrial Fibrillation: rationale and design of the ROCKET AF study. Am Heart J. 2010;159(3):340–347.e1.
18. Granger CB, Alexander JH, McMurray JJ, Lopes RD, Hylek EM, Hanna M, et al. Apixaban versus warfarin in patients with atrial fibrillation. N Engl J Med. 2011;365(11):981–92.
19. Andexxa. FDA approval letter. May 3. Available at: https://www.fda.gov/media/113954/download. Accessed June 2024.

Dental Management of Patients Taking Direct Oral Anticoagulant Drugs

24

Branislav V. Bajkin and Alison Dougall

Box 24.1 Dental Management of Patients Taking Direct Oral Anticoagulants

1. *Direct thrombin inhibitor (dabigatran)*
2. *Factor Xa inhibitors (rivaroxaban, apixaban, edoxaban)*

Oral surgery in patients taking DOAC

- Consult the patient's physician to discuss the risk of bleeding and the risk of thromboembolism
- Routine preoperative laboratory screening is usually not required
- Dental extractions, simple implant placement and other minor oral surgical procedures are considered to be safe without discontinuing DOAC
- In a case of more extensive surgery (full mouth extraction, difficult third molar surgery, periodontal surgery, soft and bone tissue augmentation procedures, orthognathic surgery etc.) temporary cessation of DOAC should be considered in consultation with patient's physician. Skipping the morning dose of DOAC taken BID (dabigatran, apixaban) or delaying the dose of DOAC taken QD (rivaroxaban, edoxaban) may be a suggested treatment option
- Treatment modification should be initiated and carefully planned by patient's physicians. It depends on the risk of the thromboembolism, procedure bleeding risk, half-live of the drug and renal function (CrCl)
- Avoid the use of the drugs that may interfere with DOAC effect

(continued)

B. V. Bajkin (✉)
University of Novi Sad, Faculty of Medicine, Dentistry Clinic of Vojvodina, Novi Sad, Serbia
e-mail: branislav.bajkin@mf.uns.ac.rs

A. Dougall
School of Dental Science, Trinity College Dublin, Dublin Dental University Hospital, Dublin, Ireland

B. V. Bajkin (ed.), *Bleeding Disorders and Dentistry*,
https://doi.org/10.1007/978-3-032-26713-9_24

Box 24.1 (continued)

- Schedule a patient at the beginning of the work week
- IANB is considered to be safe
- Use of local anesthesia with adrenalin, if not otherwise contraindicated
- Minimally traumatic surgical technique; multiple appointments may be necessary; consider carrying out the treatments in a stage manner, if possible
- Use of local hemostatic agents and measures to control oral bleeding; suturing of postextraction socket should be considered
- For pain relief use acetaminophen if not contraindicated; avoid aspirin and other NSAIDs
- Provide a patient with postoperative instructions (soft and cold diet, phone number in case of an emergency) and regular follow-up
- In a patient receiving combined DOAC and antiplatelet therapy there is a higher risk of postoperative bleeding but there is no need for cessation of either DOAC or antiplatelet therapy for simple tooth extractions and other minor oral surgical procedures

DOAC direct oral anticoagulants, *BID* twice a day, *QD* once a day, *CrCl* creatinine clearance, *IANB* inferior alveolar nerve block, *NSAIDs* nonsteroidal anti-inflammatory drugs

The main adverse effect of direct oral anticoagulants (DOACs) is bleeding, either spontaneous or due to trauma or surgery. The risk of bleeding after oral surgery in patients receiving DOACs remains an area of ongoing research. The number of such studies is lower than those related to patients on vitamin K antagonist (VKA) therapy.

In patients taking direct thrombin or FXa inhibitors, there is a risk of prolonged bleeding following tooth extraction [1]. However, interrupting DOAC therapy is associated with an increased risk of thromboembolic events [2]. Most studies and recommendations in the current literature suggest that there is no need to discontinue DOAC therapy for minor oral surgical procedures, including the extraction of up to three teeth [3–14]. The risk of bleeding following tooth extraction is estimated to be similar to or slightly lower than that in patients taking VKAs with an International Normalized Ratio (INR) within the therapeutic range [15–22]. For drugs administered once a day, some authors advocate scheduling the procedure at the time when the lowest plasma concentration of the drug is anticipated [11, 21]. The procedure should be performed as atraumatically as possible, with the use of local hemostatic measures. Careful planning of the procedure can reduce operative trauma, for example, by performing multiple tooth extractions in several visits. Laboratory testing is not routinely performed for oral surgery. Renal insufficiency prolongs the half-life of these drugs, particularly of dabigatran, and is a risk factor for postoperative bleeding [11]. In such cases, consultation with the patient's physician is mandatory.

When planning a surgical procedure associated with a higher risk of postoperative bleeding, temporary discontinuation of DOAC therapy should be carefully considered in consultation with the patient's physician. Compared with VKAs, DOACs offer several advantages for temporary therapy interruption. Following discontinuation of the therapy, the effects of these drugs subside rapidly due to their short half-life. Additionally, their effect is more rapid than that of VKAs following therapy reinitiation. Based on all of the above, it can be concluded that, when a temporary interruption of therapy is necessary, the patient may be left without anticoagulant treatment for a very short period. For DOACs administered twice a day (dabigatran and apixaban), it may be appropriate to omit the morning dose, while for DOACs taken once a day (rivaroxaban and edoxaban), a simple delay in the timing of administration may suffice. In the event of mild to moderate postoperative hemorrhage, omission of the subsequent dose may be considered [4]. Any decision regarding therapy interruption or adjustment of the dosing regimen must be made in consultation with the prescribing physician.

DOACs have significantly fewer drug interactions than VKAs. Drugs that may interact with DOACs and are used in routine dental practice should be avoided. Nonsteroidal anti-inflammatory drugs (NSAIDs), primarily acetylsalicylic acid, but also others (ibuprofen, diclofenac), can increase the risk of bleeding due to their antiplatelet effect. Paracetamol (acetaminophen) is considered the analgesic of choice for patients taking DOACs. The use of rifampicin should be avoided in patients receiving DOAC therapy. Carbamazepine may reduce plasma concentrations of DOACs, and its use requires caution or should be avoided. Dexamethasone can also decrease the effect of DOACs [4, 23].

Unlike the previously mentioned agents, some antibiotics and antifungal medications may enhance the effect of DOACs. Macrolide antibiotics such as clarithromycin and erythromycin should be avoided for this reason. Antifungal agents, such as itraconazole, ketoconazole, fluconazole, posaconazole, and voriconazole, are either contraindicated or require careful monitoring of anticoagulant therapy and potential dose adjustment [4, 23].

24.1 Dental Implant Placement in Patients Taking Direct Oral Anticoagulants

Trauma associated with implant placement is comparable to that of tooth extraction, and the risk of bleeding is therefore similar. A minimally invasive approach, such as the "flapless technique," along with the use of surgical guides, can reduce operative trauma and eliminate potential inaccuracies, thereby making the procedure safer [24, 25].

Results from most studies and recommendations in the current literature suggest that simple dental implant placement can be safely performed in patients taking DOACs without interrupting therapy [6, 26–34]. In contrast, some authors consider dental implant procedures high risk for postoperative bleeding [4] and recommend temporarily discontinuing DOAC therapy [35, 36]. Such an approach should be particularly considered in cases involving the placement of multiple implants or when a single implant placement requires a sinus lift or other extensive bone or soft tissue augmentation procedures [31, 34]. Particular caution is required during mandibular implant placement to avoid perforation of the lingual cortex and consequent bleeding into the floor of the mouth.

References

1. Bensi C, Belli S, Paradiso D, Lomurno G. Postoperative bleeding risk of direct oral anticoagulants after oral surgery procedures: a systematic review and meta-analysis. Int J Oral Maxillofac Surg. 2018;47:923–32.
2. Chan N, Sobieraj-Teague M, Eikelboom JW. Direct oral anticoagulants: evidence and unresolved issues. Lancet. 2020;396(10264):1767–76.
3. Firriolo JF, Hupp WS. Beyond warfarin: the new generation of oral anticoagulants and their implications for the management of dental patients. Oral Surg Oral Med Oral Pathol Oral Radiol. 2012;113(4):431–41.
4. Scottish Dental Clinical Effectiveness Programme. Management of dental patients taking anticoagulants or antiplatelet drugs. Dental clinical guidance. 2nd ed; 2022. Available online at: https://www.sdcep.org.uk/media/ypnl2cpz/sdcep-management-of-dental-patients-taking-anticoagulants-or-antiplatelet-drugs-2nd-edition.pdf. Accessed June 2024.
5. American Dental Association. Oral anticoagulant and antiplatelet medications and dental procedures. Available online at: https://www.ada.org/resources/research/science-and-research-institute/oral-health-topics/oral-anticoagulant-and-antiplatelet-medications-and-dental-procedures. Accessed June 2024.
6. Heidbuchel H, Verhamme P, Alings M, Antz M, Diener HC, Hacke W, Oldgren J, Sinnaeve P, Camm AJ, Kirchhof P. Updated European Heart Rhythm Association Practical Guide on the use of non-vitamin K antagonist anticoagulants in patients with non-valvular atrial fibrillation. EP Europace. 2015;17(10):1467–507.
7. Hanken H, Gröbe A, Heiland M, Smeets R, Kluwe L, Wikner J, Koehnke R, Al-Dam A, Eichhorn W. Postoperative bleeding risk for oral surgery under continued rivaroxaban anticoagulant therapy. Clin Oral Investig. 2016;20(6):1279–82.
8. Miclotte I, Vanhaverbeke M, Agbaje JO, Legrand P, Vanassche T, Verhamme P, Politis C. Pragmatic approach to manage new oral anticoagulants in patients undergoing dental extractions: a prospective case–control study. Clin Oral Investig. 2017;21(7):2183–8.
9. Morimoto Y, Yokoe C, Imai Y, Sugihara M, Futatsuki T. Tooth extraction in patients taking nonvitamin K antagonist oral anticoagulants. J Dent Sci. 2016;11:59–64.
10. Rocha A, Oliveira S, Souza A, Travassos D, Abreu L, Ribeiro D, et al. Direct oral anticoagulants in oral surgery: a prospective cohort. Minerva Stomatol. 2020;69:384–93.
11. Cocero N, Basso M, Grosso S, Carossa S. Direct oral anticoagulants and medical comorbidities in patients needing dental extractions: management of the risk of bleeding. J Oral Maxillofac Surg. 2019;77(3):463–70.
12. Miller SG, Miller CS. Direct oral anticoagulants: a retrospective study of bleeding, behavior, and documentation. Oral Dis. 2018;24(1–2):243–8.
13. Patel JP, Woolcombe SA, Patel RK, Obisesan O, Roberts LN, Bryant C, Arya R. Managing direct oral anticoagulants in patients undergoing dentoalveolar surgery. Br Dent J. 2017;222(4):245–9.
14. Durso SC. Oral manifestations of disease. In section: Disorders of eyes, ears, nose and throat. In: Harrison's principles of internal medicine. 20th ed. McGraw-Hill Education eBook; 2018. p. 219–25.

15. Healey JS, Eikelboom J, Douketis J, Wallentin L, Oldgren J, Yang S, et al. Periprocedural bleeding and thromboembolic events with dabigatran compared with warfarin: results from the Randomized Evaluation of Long-Term Anticoagulation Therapy (RELY) randomized trial. Circulation. 2012;126(3):343–8.
16. Bajkin BV, Tadic AJ, Komsic JJ, Vuckovic BA. Risk of dentoalveolar surgery postoperative bleeding in patients taking direct oral anticoagulants and vitamin K antagonists: a prospective observational study. J Craniomaxillofac Surg. 2024;52(6):772–7.
17. Johansson K, Götrick B, Holst J, Tranæus S, Naimi-Akbar A. Impact of direct oral anticoagulants on bleeding tendency and postoperative complications in oral surgery: a systematic review of controlled studies. Oral Surg Oral Med Oral Pathol Oral Radiol. 2023;135(3):333–46.
18. Berton F, Costantinides F, Rizzo R, et al. Should we fear direct oral anticoagulants more than vitamin K antagonists in simple single tooth extraction? A prospective comparative study. Clin Oral Investig. 2019;23:3183–92.
19. Brennan Y, Gu Y, Schifter M, Crowther H, Favaloro EJ, Curnow J. Dental extractions on direct oral anticoagulants vs. warfarin: the DENTST study. Res Pract Thromb Haemost. 2020;4:278–84.
20. Yoshikawa H, Yoshida M, Yasaka M, Yoshida H, Murasato Y, Fukunaga D, Shintani A, Okada Y. Safety of tooth extraction in patients receiving direct oral anticoagulant treatment versus warfarin: a prospective observation study. Int J Oral Maxillofac Surg. 2019;48(8):1102–8.
21. Mauprivez C, Khonsari RH, Razouk O, Goudot P, Lesclous P, Descroix V. Management of dental extraction in patients undergoing anticoagulant oral direct treatment: a pilot study. Oral Surg Oral Med Oral Pathol Oral Radiol. 2016;122(5):e146–55.
22. Lababidi E, Breik O, Savage J, Engelbrecht H, Kumar R, Crossley CW. Assessing an oral surgery specific protocol for patients on direct oral anticoagulants: a retrospective controlled cohort study. Int J Oral Maxillofac Surg. 2018;47(7):940–6.
23. Ferri N, Colombo E, Tenconi M, Baldessin L, Corsini A. Drug–drug interactions of direct oral anticoagulants (DOACs): from pharmacological to clinical practice. Pharmaceutics. 2022;14(6):1120.
24. Gandhi Y, Bhatavdekar N. MIDAS (Minimally Invasive Drilling And Styptic) protocol—a modified approach to treating patients under therapeutic anticoagulants. J Oral Biol Craniofac Res. 2019;9(3):208–11.
25. Al Zoman H, Al Jetaily S, Robert AA, Baskaradoss JK, Al-Suwyed A, Ciancio S, Mubarak SA. Flapless dental implant surgery for patients on oral anticoagulants—the "WarLess Procedure": a report of 2 cases. J Oral Implantol. 2013;39:264–70.
26. Gómez-Moreno G, Aguilar-Salvatierra A, Fernández-Cejas E, Delgado-Ruiz RA, Markovic A, Calvo-Guirado JL. Dental implant surgery in patients in treatment with the anticoagulant oral rivaroxaban. Clin Oral Implants Res. 2016;27(6):730–3.
27. Gómez-Moreno G, Fernández-Cejas E, Aguilar-Salvatierra A, de Carlos F, Delgado-Ruiz RA, Calvo-Guirado JL. Dental implant surgery in patients in treatment by dabigatran. Clin Oral Implants Res. 2018;29(6):644–8.
28. Clemm R, Neukam FW, Rusche B, Bauersachs A, Musazada S, Schmitt CM. Management of anticoagulated patients in implant therapy: a clinical comparative study. Clin Oral Implants Res. 2016;27(10):1274–82.
29. Zeevi I, Allon DM, Rosenfeld E, Avishai G, Gilman L, Nissan J, Chaushu G. Four-year cross-sectional study of bleeding risk in dental patients on direct oral anticoagulants. Quintessence Int. 2017;48(6):503–9.
30. Manor Y, Peleg O, Mijiritsky E, Manor A, Reiter S. A retrospective analysis of dental implantation under anticoagulant treatment. Clin Oral Investig. 2021;25(3):1001–9.
31. Dawoud BES, Kent S, Tabbenor O, George P, Dhanda J. Dental implants and risk of bleeding in patients on oral anticoagulants: a systematic review and meta-analysis. Int J Implant Dent. 2021;7(1):82.
32. Zou L, Hua L. Risk of bleeding with dental implant surgery in patients on anticoagulant or antiplatelet drugs: a systematic review and meta-analysis. Acta Odontol Scand. 2023;81(2):98–104.

33. Miziara LNB, Sendyk WR, Ortega KL, Gallottini M, Sendyk DI, Martins F. Risk of Bleeding during implant surgery in patients taking antithrombotics: a systematic review. Semin Thromb Hemost. 2021;47(6):702–8.
34. Bajkin BV, Wahl MJ, Miller CS. Dental implant surgery and risk of bleeding in patients on antithrombotic medications: a review of the literature. Oral Surg Oral Med Oral Pathol Oral Radiol. 2020;130(5):522–32.
35. Kwak EJ, Nam S, Park KM, Kim SY, Huh J, Park W. Bleeding related to dental treatment in patients taking novel oral anticoagulants (NOACs): a retrospective study. Clin Oral Investig. 2019;23(1):477–84.
36. Galletti G, Alfonsi F, Raffaele A, Valente NA, Chatelain S, Kolerman R, Cinquini C, Romeggio S, Iezzi G, Barone A. Implant placement in patients under treatment with rivaroxaban: a retrospective clinical study. Int J Environ Res Public Health. 2020;17(12):4607.

Antiplatelet Drugs

25

Branislav V. Bajkin and Ivana Urosevic

Platelets play a multifaceted role in hemostasis. By adhering to and aggregating on exposed collagen, platelets form a mechanical barrier at the site of vascular injury, accelerate the activation of coagulation factors, and promote vasoconstriction and wound healing [1]. Their function is mediated by activation of membrane receptors and complex intracellular signaling pathways (Fig. 2.1a, b).

Drugs that inhibit platelet function are known as antiplatelet agents. The major representatives of this group include acetylsalicylic acid, dipyridamole, ticlopidine, clopidogrel, prasugrel, ticagrelor, and glycoprotein IIb/IIIa antagonists (Fig. 25.1).

The most common indications for these drugs are the primary and secondary prevention of ischemic cardiovascular diseases (such as angina pectoris and myocardial infarction) and cerebrovascular diseases (including transient ischemic attack and ischemic stroke) [2–4]. When used for primary prevention of cardiovascular diseases, it is essential to weigh the benefits of this treatment against the potential risk of bleeding. Given the prevalence of these diseases, antiplatelet agents are among the most commonly prescribed medications today [5].

Because of their different mechanisms of action, the combined use of these drugs can produce a synergistic antiplatelet effect. Dual antiplatelet therapy (DAPT) most commonly involves aspirin combined with clopidogrel, prasugrel, or ticagrelor and is used in the management of acute coronary syndrome or following coronary artery stent insertion or bypass surgery [6–8]. There are no specific antagonists to reverse the effects of antiplatelet drugs, and their primary adverse effect is bleeding, which may occur spontaneously or after trauma or surgery.

B. V. Bajkin (✉)
University of Novi Sad, Faculty of Medicine, Dentistry Clinic of Vojvodina, Novi Sad, Serbia
e-mail: branislav.bajkin@mf.uns.ac.rs

I. Urosevic
University of Novi Sad, Faculty of Medicine, University Clinical Center of Vojvodina, Clinic of Hematology, Novi Sad, Serbia

B. V. Bajkin (ed.), *Bleeding Disorders and Dentistry*,
https://doi.org/10.1007/978-3-032-26713-9_25

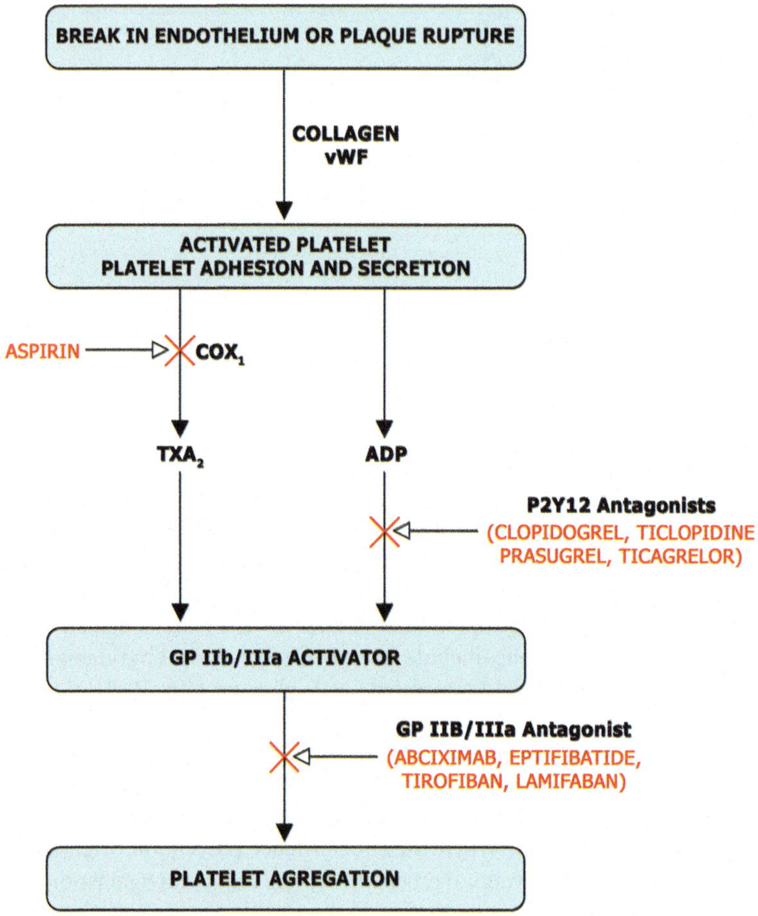

Fig. 25.1 Antiplatelet drugs: site of action

Acetylsalicylic Acid

Acetylsalicylic acid (aspirin) is an inexpensive and effective and the most commonly used antiplatelet drug. Its effect is achieved through the irreversible inactivation of cyclooxygenase (COX), an enzyme essential for the synthesis of prostaglandin H_2, a precursor of thromboxane A_2 (TXA_2) and prostacyclin (PGI_2). TXA_2 induces platelet aggregation and vasoconstriction, whereas PGI_2 has the opposite effect, inhibiting platelet aggregation and causing vasodilation (Fig. 2.2). At low doses (75–100 mg/day), aspirin selectively inhibits the synthesis of TXA_2 without significantly affecting the synthesis of PGI_2, which underlies its antiplatelet effect [1, 4, 8].

The effect of aspirin is irreversible and lasts for the lifespan of the platelet (7–10 days). Because the bone marrow continuously produces and releases new functional platelets into the bloodstream, daily aspirin administration is necessary to maintain a consistent antiplatelet effect. It is estimated that approximately

10–12% of circulating platelets are replaced daily [4]. For prophylactic use in cardiovascular diseases, aspirin is most commonly administered at doses of 100–325 mg/day [8].

The most common adverse effect of aspirin is gastrointestinal bleeding, resulting from the drug's aggressive action on the gastroduodenal mucosa. This effect is dose-dependent. There is an increased tendency toward bleeding in general, with intracranial hemorrhage being the most clinically significant, along with bleeding following invasive medical procedures. Due to the increased risk of bleeding, additional caution is required when administering DAPT or when aspirin is combined with an oral anticoagulant. It is estimated that up to one-third of patients may show "aspirin resistance," characterized by an increased tendency toward thromboembolism despite ongoing antiplatelet treatment [4, 8].

Dipyridamole

Dipyridamole (Attia®, Ofcram PR®, Persantin®) exerts both antiplatelet and vasodilatory effects. By increasing the intracellular concentration of cyclic adenosine monophosphate (cAMP) in platelets, dipyridamole inhibits platelet aggregation. It is a reversible inhibitor of the enzyme phosphodiesterase, thereby preventing degradation of cAMP. It also suppresses adenosine reuptake by inhibiting equilibrative nucleoside transporter-1 (ENT-1), which is present in various cell types, including red blood cells, platelets, endothelial cells, and cardiomyocytes. Dipyridamole also inhibits TXA_2 synthesis. The drug is rarely used as an antiplatelet agent because its antiplatelet action is weak and it may worsen exercise-induced myocardial ischemia. Dipyridamole is used in combination with acetylsalicylic acid (Asasantin®, Aggrenox®) for stroke prevention in patients with transient ischemic attack [8].

ADP Receptor Antagonists

ADP receptor antagonists, as a group of drugs, include thienopyridines and ticagrelor. These drugs are antagonists of the $P2Y_{12}$ receptor, which plays a key role in platelet activation.

Thienopyridines are selective ADP receptor/$P2Y_{12}$ antagonists that inhibit adenosine diphosphate (ADP)-mediated platelet activation. This group of drugs includes ticlopidine (Ticlid®, Ticlodix®), clopidogrel (Plavix®, Grepid®, Iscover®, Zyllt®), and prasugrel (Effient®, Prasita®). Ticlopidine is the first-generation agent in this class. Due to its toxic effects on the bone marrow and the associated risk of neutropenia and thrombotic thrombocytopenic purpura (TTP), this drug is now rarely used [4, 9].

Clopidogrel and prasugrel are prodrugs that require metabolic activation in the liver via the cytochrome P450 (CYP450) enzyme system to become pharmacologically active. Like aspirin, these agents irreversibly inhibit platelet function.

Clopidogrel belongs to the second generation of thienopyridines. Compared with ticlopidine, clopidogrel is more potent, has a more rapid onset of action, and has an improved safety profile, with a lower risk of neutropenia and thrombocytopenia. It is the most widely used agent in this class. The indications for its use are similar to those for acetylsalicylic acid. The drug is indicated for prophylactic and therapeutic use in patients with ischemic cardiovascular and cerebrovascular conditions, as well as in those with peripheral arterial disease. It can be used in patients with aspirin allergy as well. Due to the different mechanisms of action and synergistic effects, DAPT with aspirin and clopidogrel can be used and is particularly recommended following percutaneous coronary intervention. Alongside the benefits of such dual therapy, there is an increased risk of bleeding complications [4, 7–9]. The main disadvantages of clopidogrel treatment are variable absorption of the drug and individual variations in the drug response, primarily due to genetic polymorphisms of the gene coding for CYP2C19 enzyme [1, 8]. Additionally, following initiation of the therapy, the drug has a slow onset of action and a delayed offset of its effect after the interruption. The therapy typically begins with an initial dose of 300–600 mg, followed by a maintenance dose of 75 mg once a day [4, 8]. After discontinuation of the therapy, it takes 7–10 days for platelet function to be fully restored.

Prasugrel is approximately ten times more potent than clopidogrel and has a faster, more reliable antiplatelet effect due to better drug absorption. However, it has been in clinical use for a shorter period than clopidogrel. It is commonly administered as an initial dose of 60 mg, followed by a maintenance dose of 10 mg once a day. It can be used in combination with aspirin as a DAPT in patients with acute coronary syndrome and after coronary artery stent implantation [7, 8]. Due to the increased risk of bleeding, the drug is not recommended for use in patients over 75 years of age or in those with a history of cerebrovascular disease [8].

Ticagrelor (Brilinta®, Brilique®, Possia®) is an ATP analog and a reversible P2Y12 receptor antagonist that binds to a distinct site on the receptor, unlike thienopyridines. Unlike clopidogrel and prasugrel, it is not a prodrug and does not require prior activation in the liver. For this reason, it acts more rapidly than drugs administered as inactive prodrugs, with a more predictable and stronger antiplatelet effect. It can also be used in combination with aspirin as a DAPT in patients with acute coronary syndrome and after percutaneous coronary intervention and coronary stent placement [7, 8]. The therapy is initiated with a loading dose of 180 mg, followed by a maintenance dose of 90 mg twice a day.

Antagonists of Glycoprotein IIb/IIIa Receptors

Antagonists of the glycoprotein IIb/IIIa (GP IIb/IIIa) receptor include abciximab, tirofiban, and eptifibatide. These drugs inhibit the binding of von Willebrand factor (vWF) and fibrinogen to the GP IIb/IIIa complex on the platelet surface, thereby blocking the final step of platelet aggregation. These drugs are administered parenterally in acute coronary syndrome. They have an almost immediate onset of action and a dose-dependent effect. The effect of abciximab lasts 8–12 h, whereas tirofiban and eptifibatide have a duration of action of 4–8 h [10]. The main adverse effects of these drugs are bleeding and immune-mediated thrombocytopenia [8, 9]. Thrombocytopenia occurs more frequently following the administration of abciximab than with tirofiban or eptifibatide.

References

1. Baglin T. Drugs and haemostasis. In: Bennet PN, Brown MJ, Sharma P, editors. Clinical pharmacology. 11th ed. China: Churchill Livingstone Elsevier; 2012. p. 482–95.
2. Antithrombotic Trialists' Collaboration. Collaborative meta-analysis of randomised trials of antiplatelet therapy for prevention of death, myocardial infarction, and stroke in high risk patients. BMJ. 2002;324(7329):71–86.
3. Antithrombotic Trialists' (ATT) Collaboration, Baigent C, Blackwell L, Collins R, Emberson J, Godwin J, et al. Aspirin in the primary and secondary prevention of vascular disease: collaborative meta-analysis of individual participant data from randomized trials. Lancet. 2009;373(9678):1849–60.
4. Eikelboom JW, Hirsh J, Spencer FA, Baglin TP, Weitz JI. Antiplatelet drugs: antithrombotic therapy and prevention of thrombosis, 9th ed: American College of Chest Physicians Evidence-Based Clinical Practice Guidelines. Chest. 2012;141(2 Suppl):e89S–e119S.
5. Martin SS, Aday AW, Allen NB, Almarzooq ZI, Anderson CAM, Arora P, Avery CL, Baker-Smith CM, Bansal N, Beaton AZ, Commodore-Mensah Y, Currie ME, Elkind MSV, Fan W, Generoso G, Gibbs BB, Heard DG, Hiremath S, Johansen MC, Kazi DS, Ko D, Leppert MH, Magnani JW, Michos ED, Mussolino ME, Parikh NI, Perman SM, Rezk-Hanna M, Roth GA, Shah NS, Springer MV, St-Onge MP, Thacker EL, Urbut SM, Van Spall HGC, Voeks JH, Whelton SP, Wong ND, Wong SS, Yaffe K, Palaniappan LP, American Heart Association Council on Epidemiology and Prevention Statistics Committee and Stroke Statistics Committee. Heart disease and stroke statistics: a report of US and global data from the American Heart Association. Circulation. 2025;151(8):e41–e660. Epub 2025 Jan 27. Erratum in: Circulation. 2025;151(25):e1096.
6. Grines CL, Bonow RO, Casey DE Jr, Gardner TJ, Lockhart PB, Moliterno DJ, et al. Prevention of premature discontinuation of dual antiplatelet therapy in patients with coronary artery stents: a science advisory from the American Heart Association, American College of Cardiology, Society for Cardiovascular Angiography and Interventions, American College of Surgeons, and American Dental Association, with representation from the American College of Physicians. Circulation. 2007;115(6):813–8.
7. Scottish Dental Clinical Effectiveness Programme. Management of dental patients taking anticoagulants or antiplatelet drugs. Dental Clinical Guidance. 2nd ed. 2022. Available online at: https://www.sdcep.org.uk/media/ypnl2cpz/sdcep-management-of-dental-patients-taking-anticoagulants-or-antiplatelet-drugs-2nd-edition.pdf. Accessed June 2024.
8. Weitz JI. Antiplatelet, anticoagulant, and fibrinolytic drugs. In section: disorders of hemostasis. In: Harrison's principles of internal medicine. 20th ed. McGraw-Hill Education eBook; 2018. p. 843–58.
9. Scully C. Haemathology. In: Scully's medical problems in dentistry. 7th ed. Churchill Livingstone: Elsevier; 2014. p. 212–75.
10. Little JW, Miller CS, Rhodus NL. Acquired bleeding and hypercoagulable disorders. In: Little and Falace's dental management of the medically compromised patient. 8th ed. St. Louis: Elsevier; 2018. p. 428–56.

Dental Management of Patients Taking Antiplatelet Medications

26

Branislav V. Bajkin and Alison Dougall

Box 26.1 Dental Management of Patients Taking Antiplatelet Medications

Antiplatelet drugs

1. Acetylsalicylic acid
2. Dipyridamole
3. ADP receptor antagonists: thienopyridines (ticlopidine, clopidogrel, prasugrel), ticagrelor
4. Glycoprotein IIb/IIIa receptor antagonists (abciximab, tirofiban, lamifiban, eptifibatide)

Oral surgery in patients taking antiplatelet drugs

- Consult the patient's physician to discuss the risk of bleeding and the risk of thromboembolism
- Routine preoperative laboratory screening is usually not required
- Dental extractions, simple implant placement, and other minor oral surgical procedures are considered to be safe without discontinuing single or dual antiplatelet therapy
- In a case of more extensive surgery (full mouth extraction, difficult third molar surgery, periodontal surgery, soft and bone tissue augmentation procedures, orthognathic surgery, etc.), temporary cessation of antiplatelet

(continued)

B. V. Bajkin (✉)
University of Novi Sad, Faculty of Medicine, Dentistry Clinic of Vojvodina, Novi Sad, Serbia
e-mail: branislav.bajkin@mf.uns.ac.rs

A. Dougall
School of Dental Science, Trinity College Dublin, Dublin Dental University Hospital, Dublin, Ireland

B. V. Bajkin (ed.), *Bleeding Disorders and Dentistry*,
https://doi.org/10.1007/978-3-032-26713-9_26

Box 26.1 (continued)

therapy may be considered in consultation with patient's physician. Treatment modification should be initiated and carefully planned by patient's physicians
- In a patient receiving combined VKA and antiplatelet therapy, there is a higher risk of postoperative bleeding, but there is no need for cessation of either VKA or antiplatelet therapy for simple tooth extractions and other minor oral surgical procedures, if INR is within therapeutic range and local hemostasis measures are used
- In a patient receiving combined DOACs and antiplatelet therapy, there is a higher risk of postoperative bleeding, but there is no need for cessation of either DOACs or antiplatelet therapy for simple tooth extractions and other minor oral surgical procedures
- Schedule a patient at the beginning of the work week
- IANB is considered to be safe
- Use of local anesthesia with adrenalin, if not otherwise contraindicated
- Minimally traumatic surgical technique; multiple appointments may be necessary; consider carrying out the treatments in a stage manner, if possible
- Use of local hemostatic agents and measures to control oral bleeding; suturing of postextraction socket should be considered
- For pain relief, use acetaminophen if not contraindicated; avoid NSAIDs
- Provide a patient with postoperative instructions (soft and cold diet, phone number in case of an emergency) and regular follow-up

ADP adenosine diphosphate, *VKA* vitamin K antagonists, *INR* International Normalized Ratio, *IANB* inferior alveolar nerve block, *DOACs* direct oral anticoagulants, *NSAIDs* nonsteroidal anti-inflammatory drugs

For patients who are taking any type of antithrombotic medication and require oral surgery, a clear decision must be made whether to continue the therapy, which is associated with an increased risk of prolonged, excessive bleeding during and after the procedure, or to discontinue the treatment, which carries the risk of a thromboembolic event.

In the past, patients were generally advised to stop taking antiplatelet drugs for several days before the procedure. However, this approach may have increased the risk of thromboembolic complications [1–4]. The literature documents thromboembolic events occurring after the interruption of antiplatelet therapy for dental interventions [5]. By contrast, the literature does not report cases of severe bleeding following oral surgical procedures in patients taking antiplatelet drugs. If postoperative bleeding occurs, it is typically easily controlled with local hemostatic measures [6].

Most studies suggest that discontinuation of antiplatelet therapy is not necessary for tooth extractions or other oral surgical interventions [7–12]. The risk of bleeding following tooth extraction in patients on aspirin therapy is higher compared to those who either do not take the drug or have temporarily stopped using it; however, postoperative bleeding is generally not severe and can be effectively managed with local hemostatic measures [5, 13–15]. Based on the latest research findings, recommendations are that antiplatelet therapy should not be discontinued prior to oral surgical procedures, including tooth extractions [16–21].

Patients receiving antiplatelet therapy may have a prolonged bleeding time (BT). However, this test is not considered a reliable or clinically valid predictor of hemorrhagic risk following oral surgical procedures. Laboratory tests for platelet function assessment (such as platelet aggregation assays) are more sensitive but are not routinely used preoperatively [11]. Therefore, in patients receiving antiplatelet therapy, laboratory testing prior to oral surgical procedures is not recommended.

Nonsteroidal anti-inflammatory drugs (NSAIDs) also have antiplatelet effects by inhibiting platelet cyclooxygenase and blocking thromboxane A_2 (TXA_2) synthesis. These drugs reversibly affect platelet function by interfering with TXA_2-mediated platelet aggregation. The effect of NSAIDs on platelets is dose-dependent and influenced by plasma concentration and half-life. Dose adjustment of these drugs is not required prior to invasive dental procedures. Given NSAIDs' aggressive effects on the gastric mucosa, paracetamol is the analgesic of choice following oral surgical procedures in patients taking antiplatelet drugs.

26.1 Dental Implant Placement in Patients Taking Antiplatelet Medications

The trauma associated with dental implant placement is similar to that caused by tooth extraction. However, implant procedures do not involve only implant placement but often include bone augmentation and manipulation of soft tissues around the dental implant. In addition to their complexity and sensitivity, these procedures involve more extensive tissue manipulation and, consequently, greater surgical trauma.

Simple implant placement does not require interruption of antiplatelet therapy; however, careful procedural planning and the use of local hemostatic measures are essential [22–29].

Special caution is required when placing implants in high-risk regions, such as the anterior mandible, where perforation of the lingual cortical plate and injury to sublingual blood vessels can result in severe hemorrhage into the floor of the mouth. A minimally invasive approach, such as flapless implant placement when indicated, is particularly important, as is the use of surgical guides, which can reduce potential inaccuracies and thereby enhance the safety of the procedure [30, 31]. In cases involving more invasive procedures within the field of dental implantology, it is necessary to collaborate with the patient's physician to determine the safest treatment approach. This includes deciding whether to continue or temporarily interrupt antiplatelet therapy, based on a thorough risk assessment that balances the potential for bleeding against the risk of thromboembolic complications.

26.2 Oral Surgery in Patients Taking Dual Antiplatelet Therapy

Because these drugs have different mechanisms of action, dual antiplatelet therapy can be used. The primary indications for DAPT are post-percutaneous coronary intervention with stent placement and the management of acute coronary syndrome. The most commonly used DAPT is the combination of aspirin and clopidogrel. However, combinations of aspirin with other P2Y12 inhibitors, such as ticagrelor or prasugrel, are also employed. DAPT is indicated for up to 12 months following coronary stent implantation, after which treatment is continued with a single antiplatelet agent [32].

Elective surgical procedures are generally recommended to be deferred following an acute coronary syndrome and within the first year after coronary stent implantation, whenever clinically feasible [33]. The concomitant use of two antiplatelet agents increases the risk of bleeding, but premature discontinuation of either agent also carries significant thromboembolic risks. Premature discontinuation of antiplatelet therapy has been identified as a leading risk factor for stent thrombosis [18]. Temporary discontinuation of antiplatelet therapy for dental procedures is not recommended, and consultation with the cardiologist is strongly recommended [1, 18, 34].

The risk of bleeding during and after oral surgical procedures is expected to be higher in patients on dual antiplatelet therapy than in those taking a single agent from this group or those not receiving antiplatelet therapy. However, research findings indicate that this risk is not very high, so that postoperative bleeding can be effectively controlled with local hemostatic measures [15, 35–39]. Consequently, temporary discontinuation of DAPT is not recommended for tooth extractions or other minor oral surgical procedures [16, 17].

Concomitant use of oral anticoagulants and antiplatelet agents may be indicated in certain clinical scenarios (see Sect. 22.4).

References

1. Biondi-Zoccai GG, Lotrionte M, Agostoni P, Abbate A, Fusaro M, Burzotta F, et al. A systematic review and meta-analysis on the hazards of discontinuing or not adhering to aspirin among 50,279 patients at risk for coronary artery disease. Eur Heart J. 2006;27(22):2667–74.
2. Burger W, Chemnitius JM, Kneissl GD, Rücker G. Low-dose aspirin for secondary cardiovascular prevention – cardiovascular risks after its perioperative withdrawal versus bleeding risks with its continuation - review and meta-analysis. J Intern Med. 2005;257(5):399–414.
3. Maulaz AB, Bezerra DC, Michel P, Bogousslavsky J. Effect of discontinuing aspirin therapy on the risk of brain ischemic stroke. Arch Neurol. 2005;62(8):1217–20.
4. Ferrari E, Benhamou M, Cerboni P, Marcel B. Coronary syndromes following aspirin withdrawal: a special risk for late stent thrombosis. J Am Coll Cardiol. 2005;45(3):456–9.
5. Wahl MJ. Dental surgery and antiplatelet agents: bleed or die. Am J Med. 2014;127(4):260–7.
6. Scully C. Haemathology. In: Scully's medical problems in dentistry. 7th ed. Churchill Livingstone: Elsevier; 2014. p. 212–75.
7. Ardekian L, Gaspar R, Peled M, Brener B, Laufer D. Does low-dose aspirin therapy complicate oral surgical procedures? J Am Dent Assoc. 2000;131(3):331–5.

8. Brennan MT, Valerin MA, Noll JL, Napeñas JJ, Kent ML, Fox PC, et al. Aspirin use and post-operative bleeding from dental extractions. J Dent Res. 2008;87(8):740–4.
9. Krishnan B, Shenoy NA, Alexander M. Exodontia and antiplatelet therapy. J Oral Maxillofac Surg. 2008;66:2063–6.
10. Morimoto Y, Niwa H, Minematsu K. Risk factors affecting postoperative hemorrhage after tooth extraction in patients receiving oral antithrombotic therapy. J Oral Maxillofac Surg. 2011;69(6):1550–6.
11. Nagao Y, Masuda R, Ando A, Nonaka M, Nishimura A, Goto K, et al. Whole blood platelet aggregation test and prediction of hemostatic difficulty after tooth extraction in patients receiving antiplatelet therapy. Clin Appl Thromb Hemost. 2018;24(1):151–6.
12. Omar HR, Socias SM, Powless RA, Sprenker C, Karinoski R, Mangar D, et al. Clopidogrel is not associated with increased bleeding complications after full mouth extraction: a retrospective study. J Am Dent Assoc. 2015;146(5):303–9.
13. Zhao B, Wang P, Dong Y, Zhu Y. Should aspirin be stopped before tooth extraction? A meta-analysis. Oral Surg Oral Med Oral Pathol Oral Radiol. 2015;119:522–30.
14. Wahl MJ. Perioperative management of dental patients on antiplatelet medications. In: Szumita RP, Szumita PM, editors. Hemostasis in dentistry. Cham: Springer; 2018. p. 125–41.
15. Napeñas JJ, Oost FC, DeGroot A, Loven B, Hong CH, Brennan MT, Lockhart PB, van Diermen DE. Review of postoperative bleeding risk in dental patients on antiplatelet therapy. Oral Surg Oral Med Oral Pathol Oral Radiol. 2013;115(4):491–9.
16. Scottish Dental Clinical Effectiveness Programme. Management of dental patients taking anticoagulants or antiplatelet drugs. Dental Clinical Guidance. 2nd ed. 2022. Available online at: https://www.sdcep.org.uk/media/ypnl2cpz/sdcep-management-of-dental-patients-taking-anticoagulants-or-antiplatelet-drugs-2nd-edition.pdf. Accessed June 2024.
17. American Dental Association. Oral anticoagulant and antiplatelet medications and dental procedures. Available online at: https://www.ada.org/resources/research/science-and-research-institute/oral-health-topics/oral-anticoagulant-and-antiplatelet-medications-and-dental-procedures. Accessed June 2024.
18. Grines CL, Bonow RO, Casey DE Jr, Gardner TJ, Lockhart PB, Moliterno DJ, O'Gara P, Whitlow P, American Heart Association; American College of Cardiology; Society for Cardiovascular Angiography and Interventions; American College of Surgeons; American Dental Association; American College of Physicians. Prevention of premature discontinuation of dual antiplatelet therapy in patients with coronary artery stents: a science advisory from the American Heart Association, American College of Cardiology, Society for Cardiovascular Angiography and Interventions, American College of Surgeons, and American Dental Association, with representation from the American College of Physicians. J Am Dent Assoc. 2007;138(5):652–5.
19. Douketis JD, Spyropoulos AC, Spencer FA, Mayr M, Jaffer AK, Eckman MH, et al. Perioperative management of antithrombotic therapy: antithrombotic therapy and prevention of thrombosis, 9th ed: American College of Chest Physicians Evidence-Based Clinical Practice Guidelines. Chest. 2012;141(2 Suppl):e326S–50S.
20. Armstrong MJ, Gronseth G, Anderson DC, Biller J, Cucchiara B, Dafer R, et al. Summary of evidence-based guideline: periprocedural management of antithrombotic medications in patients with ischemic cerebrovascular disease. Report of the Guideline Development Subcommittee of the American Academy of Neurology. Neurology. 2013;80(22):2065–9.
21. Durso SC. Oral manifestations of disease. In section: disorders of eyes, ears, nose and throat. In: Harrison's principles of internal medicine. 20th ed. McGraw-Hill Education eBook; 2018. p. 219–25.
22. Tabrizi R, Khaheshi I, Hoseinzadeh A, Rezvanpour B, Shafie S. Do antiplatelet drugs increase the risk of bleeding after dental implant surgery? A case-and-crossover study. J Oral Maxillofac Surg. 2018;76(10):2092–6.
23. Broekema FI, van Minnen B, Jansma J, Bos RRM. Risk of bleeding after dentoalveolar surgery in patients taking anticoagulants. Br J Oral Maxillofac Surg. 2014;52(3):e15–9.

24. Clemm R, Neukam FW, Rusche B, Bauersachs A, Musazada S, Schmitt CM. Management of anticoagulated patients in implant therapy: a clinical comparative study. Clin Oral Implants Res. 2016;27(10):1274–82.
25. Rubino RT, Dawson DR 3rd, Kryscio RJ, Al-Sabbagh M, Miller CS. Postoperative bleeding associated with antiplatelet and anticoagulant drugs: a retrospective study. Oral Surg Oral Med Oral Pathol Oral Radiol. 2019;128(3):243–9.
26. Kaura S, Rai R, Satia G, Budhiraja N, Mohan B. Assessment of bleeding in patients on antiplatelets undergoing dental implants. J Maxillofac Oral Surg. 2022;21(1):260–4.
27. Manor Y, Peleg O, Mijiritsky E, Manor A, Reiter S. A retrospective analysis of dental implantation under anticoagulant treatment. Clin Oral Investig. 2021;25(3):1001–9.
28. Buchbender M, Schlee N, Kesting MR, Grimm J, Fehlhofer J, Rau A. A prospective comparative study to assess the risk of postoperative bleeding after dental surgery while on medication with direct oral anticoagulants, antiplatelet agents, or vitamin K antagonists. BMC Oral Health. 2021;21(1):504.
29. Bajkin BV, Wahl MJ, Miller CS. Dental implant surgery and risk of bleeding in patients on antithrombotic medications: a review of the literature. Oral Surg Oral Med Oral Pathol Oral Radiol. 2020;130(5):522–32.
30. Gandhi Y, Bhatavdekar N. MIDAS (Minimally Invasive Drilling And Styptic) protocol - a modified approach to treating patients under therapeutic anticoagulants. J Oral Biol Craniofac Res. 2019;9(3):208–11.
31. Al Zoman H, Al Jetaily S, Robert AA, Baskaradoss JK, Al-Suwyed A, Ciancio S, Mubarak SA. Flapless dental implant surgery for patients on oral anticoagulants—the "WarLess Procedure": a report of 2 cases. J Oral Implantol. 2013;39:264–70.
32. Bittl JA, Baber U, Bradley SM, Wijeysundera DN. Duration of dual antiplatelet therapy: a systematic review for the 2016 ACC/AHA guideline focused update on duration of dual antiplatelet therapy in patients with coronary artery disease: a report of the American College of Cardiology/American Heart Association Task Force on Clinical Practice Guidelines. J Am Coll Cardiol. 2016;68(10):1116–39.
33. Little JW, Miller CS, Rhodus NL. Acquired bleeding and hypercoagulable disorders. In: Little and Falace's dental management of the medically compromised patient. 9th ed. St. Louis: Elsevier; 2018. p. 428–56.
34. Mahmood H, Siddique I, McKechnie A. Antiplatelet drugs: a review of pharmacology and the perioperative management of patients in oral and maxillofacial surgery. Ann R Coll Surg Engl. 2020;102(1):1–5.
35. Bajkin BV, Urosevic IM, Stankov KM, Petrovic BB, Bajkin IA. Dental extractions and risk of bleeding in patients taking single and dual anti platelet treatment. Br J Oral Maxillofac Surg. 2015;53(1):39–43.
36. Park M, Her S, Kwon JB, Lee JB, Choi M, Cho JS, et al. Safety of dental extractions in coronary drug-eluting stenting patients without stopping multiple antiplatelet agents. Clin Cardiol. 2012;35(4):225–30.
37. Lillis T, Ziakas A, Koskinas K, Tsirlis A, Giannoglou G. Safety of dentalextractions during uninterrupted single or dual antiplatelet treatment. Am J Cardiol. 2011;108(7):964–7.
38. Sadeghi-Ghahrody M, Yousefi-Malekshah SH, Karimi-Sari H, Yazdanpanah H, Rezaee-Zavareh MS, Yavarahmadi M. Bleeding after tooth extraction in patients taking aspirin and clopidogrel (Plavix®) compared with healthy controls. Br J Oral Maxillofac Surg. 2016;54(5):568–72.
39. Ockerman A, Bornstein MM, Leung YY, Li SKY, Politis C, Jacobs R. Incidence of bleeding after minor oral surgery in patients on dual antiplatelet therapy: a systematic review and meta-analysis. Int J Oral Maxillofac Surg. 2020;49(1):90–8.

Part VI

Local Hemostasis in Dentistry

Local Hemostatic Agents and Measures 27

Branislav V. Bajkin and Alison Dougall

Oral surgical interventions have specific considerations for the prevention and management of postoperative bleeding. The likelihood of injury to major blood vessels is low, and postoperative bleeding is typically readily diagnosed and effectively controlled with local hemostatic agents and measures. Saliva has fibrinolytic properties, which in patients with a tendency to bleed, such as persons with hemophilia, may lead to the formation of an unstable blood clot and result in bleeding that can occur several days after the procedure.

Bleeding following oral surgical procedures may have a local cause, result from impaired hemostatic function, or be related to anticoagulant and antiplatelet therapy. It is critical to identify and eliminate the local cause of bleeding (Figs. 1.7a, b and 1.8). Local hemostatic measures and topical hemostatic agents are used to control intraoperative bleeding and prevent postoperative hemorrhage. Local hemostatic measures include common procedures routinely performed after tooth extraction, such as superficial wound compression with gauze, as well as the use of various topical hemostatic agents and specific techniques for bleeding control. Effective local hemostasis during the procedure improves visibility of the surgical field, reduces procedure duration, and decreases the risk of postoperative complications.

B. V. Bajkin (✉)
University of Novi Sad, Faculty of Medicine, Dentistry Clinic of Vojvodina, Novi Sad, Serbia
e-mail: branislav.bajkin@mf.uns.ac.rs

A. Dougall
School of Dental Science, Trinity College Dublin, Dublin Dental University Hospital, Dublin, Ireland

B. V. Bajkin (ed.), *Bleeding Disorders and Dentistry*,
https://doi.org/10.1007/978-3-032-26713-9_27

27.1 Local Hemostatic Agents

Local hemostatics are agents applied directly to the bleeding site to promote cessation of bleeding. Local hemostatics can be classified into the following [1]:

- Agents that cause vasoconstriction and promote platelet aggregation (adrenaline, vasopressin, desmopressin, terlipressin, ornipressin, pituitrin)
- Agents that induce the transition of blood proteins into a solid state and reduce vascular permeability by protein denaturation (3% hydrogen, ferric chloride, ferric sulfate, silver nitrate, aluminum chloride, and others)
- Agents that stimulate the adhesion and aggregation of formed blood elements and accelerate fibrin formation (collagen products, gelatin, oxidized regenerated cellulose, chitosan)
- Coagulation factors (thrombin, fibrin glue)
- Antifibrinolytics (tranexamic acid, epsilon-aminocaproic acid, aprotinin)
- Combined agents (combination of several local hemostatics or local hemostatics with antibiotics or cytostatics)

According to the mechanism of action, local hemostatic agents can be further classified into the following [2–4]:

- Passive local hemostatic agents with nonspecific action on the coagulation cascade (collagen, gelatin, oxidized regenerated cellulose, chitosan); these agents are not biologically active. They primarily provide a mechanical matrix for platelet adhesion and aggregation.
- Active local hemostatic agents with specific action on the coagulation cascade (fibrin glue, thrombin); these agents are effective in cases of impaired coagulation.

A broader classification, based on the mechanism of action, categorizes local hemostatic agents into the following groups [5–7]:

- Mechanical or passive (bone wax, gelatin, collagen, oxidized regenerated cellulose, polysaccharide hemospheres),
- Active (fibrin glue, thrombin)
- Liquid (agents that represent a combination, most commonly of thrombin and gelatin)
- Adhesives (glues) that can be synthetic (cyanoacrylate or polyethylene glycol glue) and semisynthetic (glutaraldehyde-albumin-based glue)

Local hemostatics can also be classified into natural agents, which may be of plant (oxidized regenerated cellulose), animal (gelatin, collagen, thrombin, chitosan), or human origin (fibrin glue, thrombin), semisynthetic (glutaraldehyde-albumin), and synthetic preparations (cyanoacrylate glue, antifibrinolytics).

Before using any of these agents, their potential limitations and drawbacks should be considered. Fibrin glue is expensive, and because it contains human-derived components, the risk of viral transmission cannot be completely excluded, although the components undergo viral inactivation during preparation [8]. Animal-derived preparations carry a potential risk of allergic reactions. Antifibrinolytics in the form of mouthwash solutions primarily act locally on the surface of the coagulum and have no effect on bleeding that occurs deeper in the tissue. Additionally, residual components of local hemostatic agents that have not undergone spontaneous resorption may lead to infection, inflammation, and delayed wound healing.

The use of local hemostatic agents is of undeniable importance following tooth extraction in patients with hemostatic disorders [9]. The results of studies conducted in patients undergoing anticoagulant therapy who required tooth extraction have not shown that any local hemostatic agent is superior to others [10, 11]. The most commonly used local hemostatic agents in dentistry are presented in Table 27.1.

The ideal local hemostatic agent should be biocompatible, safe, and easy to use, have an almost immediate effect, and be cost-effective. There is no local hemostatic agent that fully meets all of these criteria. Therefore, new agents are being developed, either as entirely novel local hemostatics, as combinations of two or more

Table 27.1 Local hemostatic agents most commonly used in dentistry

Agents	Most common form	Indication for use	Advantages	Limitations
Gelatin products	Sponges	For mild bleeding	Easy to use Cheap Can be used with thrombin	Stick to instruments Prone to infection
Collagen products	Sponges Dressings	For mild to moderate bleeding	Easy to use Do not stick to instruments Can be shaped according to intended use	More expensive compared to gelatin-based products
Oxidized regenerated cellulose	Mesh Powder	For moderate to severe bleeding Useful to control bleeding when other agents are ineffective	Easy to use Considered to be absolutely safe Antibacterial activity Can be used with antifibrinolytics	May cause "foreign-body" reaction Cannot be used with thrombin due to its inactivation May cause nerve injury
Chitosan	Dressing	For moderate bleeding Can be placed in extraction sockets and to cover oral wounds	Easy to use Considered to be absolutely safe Self-adhesive Relieves pain	Poor solubility May cause allergic reaction Certain physical properties such as rigidity

(continued)

Table 27.1 (continued)

Agents	Most common form	Indication for use	Advantages	Limitations
Thrombin	Powder	For severe bleeding Can be dissolved in sterile saline before use	Easy to use Can be used in combination with other agents, usually gelatin Potent hemostatic agent	Rarely used alone Animal products may cause allergic reaction Human products may pose risk of viral transmission
Fibrin glue	Two-component system with double-syringe applicator	For severe bleeding Can be placed in extraction sockets or to cover oral wounds and stiches	Easy to use Facilitates wound healing Proven efficacy in persons with hemophilia Potent hemostatic agent	Expensive Risk of viral transmission due to human components Should not be routinely used in persons with hemophilia who have been treated only with recombinant blood factors
Antifibrinolytics	Tablets Ampoules Mouthwash solution Paste	Local use, either applied directly in the wound, via saturated gaze, or in the form of mouthwash solution	Cheap Useful to control mucosal bleeding in persons with hemophilia and von Willebrand disease	If used in the form of mouthwash solution, it acts only superficially on the clot If used systemically, no effect on salivary fibrinolytic activity

already available agents, or by applying new technologies to obtain preparations with improved quality [4, 7].

Gelatin

Gelatin-based agents (Gelfoam®, Gelatamp®, Gelitaspon®, Gelastip®, Gelopack®, Spongostan®, and others) are most commonly used as sterile resorbable sponges that are easily applied to the extraction socket. There are also agents in powder and gel forms. These agents consist of purified gelatin of animal origin, most commonly derived from bovine or porcine sources. Following application to the wound, gelatin sponges absorb blood plasma and swell, thereby providing a mechanical matrix for platelet adhesion and aggregation and facilitating contact activation of coagulation. Gelatin-based agents can absorb blood plasma up to approximately 40 times their own weight. Prior to application, the wound should be dried, as the sponge tends to adhere to instruments in contact with blood. The sponge should not be compressed before insertion (Fig. 27.1a–e). Compression of the sponge disrupts its porous structure and reduces its capacity to absorb blood. Gelatin undergoes hydrolytic degradation and is resorbed over a period of 4–6 weeks.

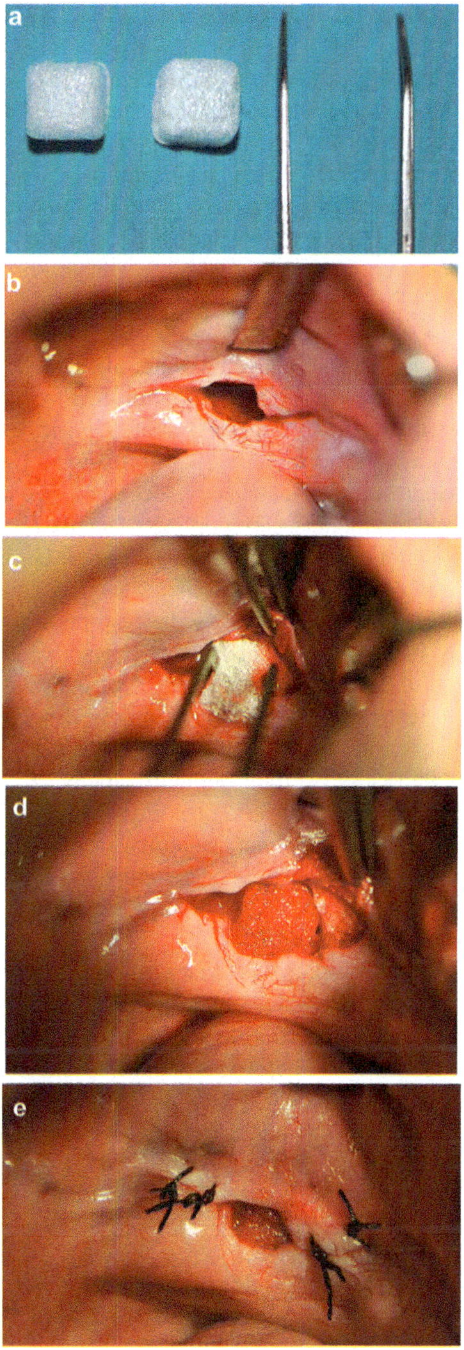

Fig. 27.1 (a–e) Application of a gelatin sponge following surgical extraction of the mandibular third molar in a patient receiving antiplatelet therapy

Gelatin-based agents are used for mild bleeding, which limits their use. Their efficacy can be improved when combined with other topical hemostatic agents. Thrombin is most commonly combined with the gelatin matrix (Floseal®, Surgiflo®). A potential limitation is that gelatin-based agents may serve as a medium for microbial growth. For this reason, some agents include antimicrobial additives. Furthermore, they may contribute to delayed wound healing because of slow resorption and the potential to elicit a foreign body reaction. Gelatin-based agents should not be applied to infected areas or in proximity to nerves, as swelling may lead to nerve compression [2, 4, 6].

Collagen Products

Microfibrillar collagen was introduced as a local hemostatic agent in the 1970s, and its effectiveness has been confirmed by numerous studies [12]. As a local hemostatic agent, collagen is available in various forms, including powder, sponge, and membrane (Avitene®, Ultrafoam®, Colla-Cote®, CollaTape®, CollaPlug®, Hemocollagen®, Helistat®, Helitene®, Instat®, and others). These agents are of animal origin, most commonly derived from bovine sources. Collagen primarily affects platelet activation and aggregation and facilitates activation of the intrinsic coagulation pathway. Given its mechanism of action, it may be less effective in patients with thrombocytopenia. The resorption period of these agents is approximately 8–10 weeks. In dental practice, resorbable collagen sponges are most commonly used. Collagen sponges can be cut and shaped as needed. They are easily applied to the extraction socket, which must be dried beforehand, and adhere well to the bleeding surface (Fig. 27.2a, b). Compared to gelatin-based agents, collagen products exhibit less swelling, act more rapidly, are more effective, and can be used in cases of moderate to severe bleeding. Although rare, allergic reactions to collagen may occur. The placement of collagen in infected areas should be avoided, as these agents do not possess bactericidal properties [4, 6, 7].

Oxidized Cellulose

Local hemostatics based on cellulose (Surgicel®, Resorcell®, Oxycell®, and others) are plant-derived agents composed of oxidized regenerated cellulose (ORC), with organized fibers before oxidation, or non-regenerated cellulose (ONRC), with unorganized fibers before oxidation. ONRC may be more effective, but it is harder to handle, which is why ORC is used far more frequently. The mechanism of action of ORC is not fully clarified, but it is believed to have a more physical than physiological effect on blood coagulation. ORC most commonly comes in the form of a sterile absorbable knitted fabric that swells upon contact with blood and turns into a brownish gelatinous mass, creating pressure and thereby mechanically stopping the bleeding (Fig. 27.3a–d). It also provides a matrix for platelet adhesion and aggregation. Furthermore, it is believed that, due to its low pH value, cellulose causes contraction of small blood vessels, protein denaturation, and contact activation of coagulation. Due to its low pH value, ORC has a bactericidal effect, so there is no tendency for infection of the surgical wound after the application of this hemostatic agent. For the same reason, it can cause chemical damage to peripheral nerves, so

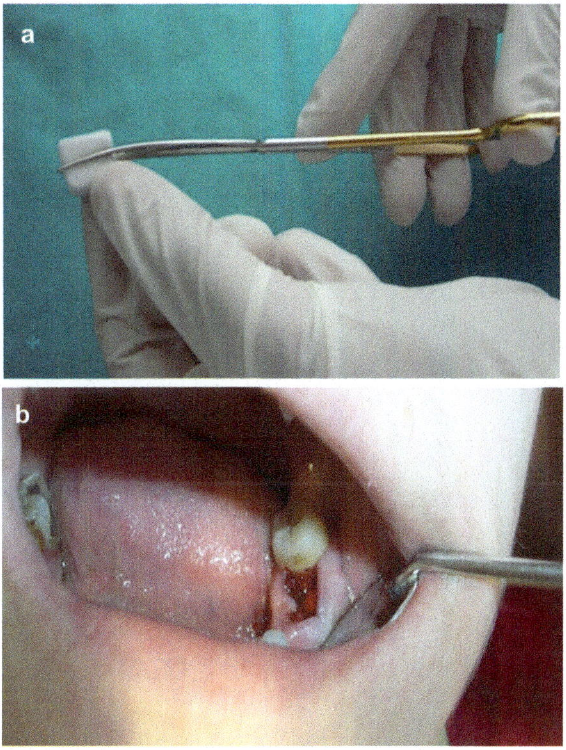

Fig. 27.2 (a, b) Application of a resorbable collagen sponge following tooth extraction in a patient receiving vitamin K antagonist therapy

the agent should not be placed near them. This primarily refers to the inferior alveolar nerve and the mental nerve in oral surgery. It inactivates thrombin, so these two preparations should not be used together. It can be used in combination with antifibrinolytics. It is absorbed by hydrolysis over a period of 4–8 weeks and therefore can be left in the wound or removed after bleeding stops. The biodegradability of the material depends on the amount applied, so it is recommended to remove any excess material. Larger amounts of the material may remain unabsorbed, cause a foreign body-type reaction, and require reoperation [4, 6, 7, 13].

ORC is one of the most commonly used local hemostatic agents in dentistry and can be used in cases of moderate to severe bleeding. For use in dentistry, ORC is also available as a powder and as pellets made of cellulose fibers (Fig. 27.4a–c), which can be useful for controlling bleeding from the gingiva and periodontium.

Other Plant-Based Local Hemostatic Agents

The advantage of plant-based local hemostatic agents over animal- and human-derived products is that their use carries no theoretical risk of transmitting viral or prion diseases. Therefore, these products are considered absolutely safe. In addition to cellulose-based agents, which are most commonly used, other plant-derived agents are also available in some countries. One of them is Ankaferd Blood Stopper®, a local hemostatic agent derived from five types of plants. It is commercially

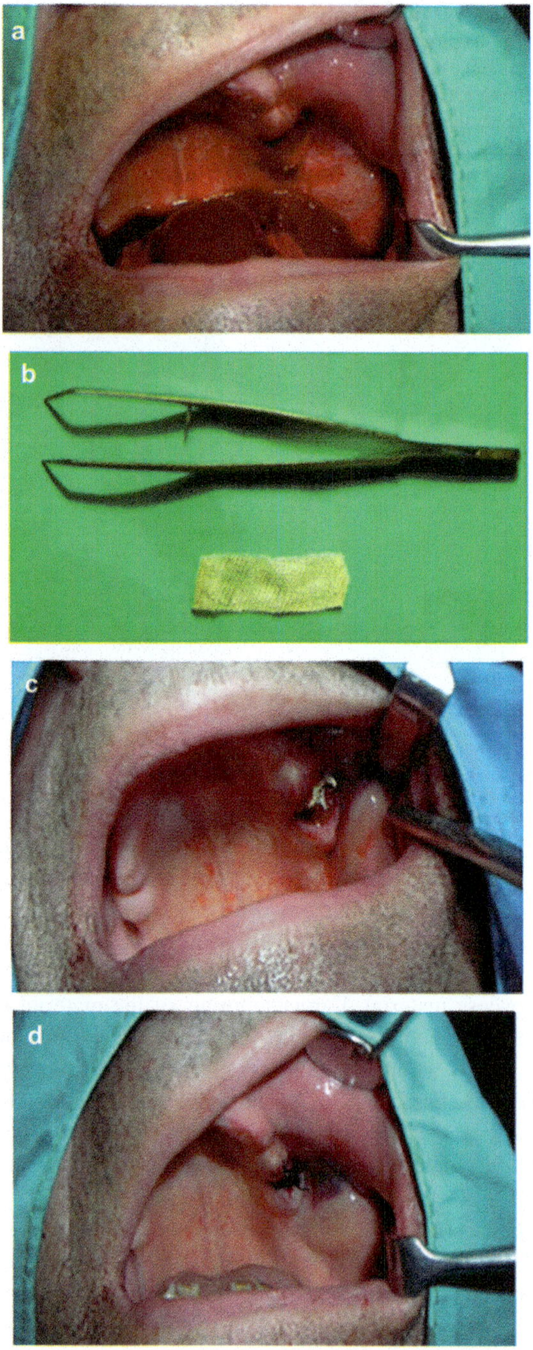

Fig. 27.3 (**a**–**d**) Use of oxidized regenerated cellulose in the management of post-extraction bleeding

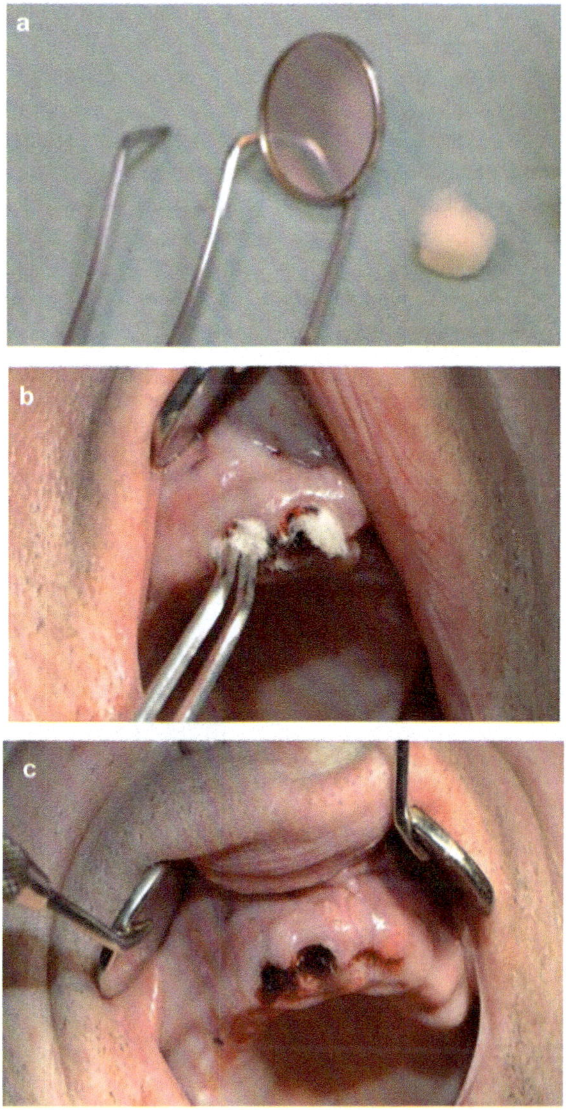

Fig. 27.4 (a–c) Use of oxidized regenerated cellulose in the form of pellets in the management of post-extraction bleeding

available in the form of ampoules, wet tampons, and sprays. After local application, it forms a protein network that accelerates erythrocyte aggregation. The number of studies regarding the use of this agent for oral surgery is limited. Several studies have shown its efficacy in patients on anticoagulant therapy [14] and in persons with hemophilia who required tooth extraction [15].

Chitosan

Chitosan (HemCon®, Celox®, and others) is a derivative of chitin. It is a copolymer of glucosamine and N-acetylglucosamine units. It is a biocompatible, naturally positively charged biopolymer found in the exoskeletons of crustaceans, which are primarily composed of chitin. Chitosan is an insoluble dietary fiber produced by deacetylation after removing proteins and calcium from chitin, so it does not contain animal proteins. Its effect is achieved through the reaction of its positively charged molecules with negatively charged membranes, primarily those of erythrocytes, forming a viscous clot that facilitates platelet aggregation, initiates the hemostatic mechanism, and promotes wound closure. The advantages of chitosan are that this local hemostatic agent is adhesive, can reduce pain by protecting the wound from irritation, accelerates wound healing, possesses bacteriostatic properties, and is resorbed within a few days after use (Fig. 27.5a–c) [1, 4, 16]. Chitosan has proven to be an effective hemostatic agent after tooth extraction in patients taking anticoagulant and antiplatelet medications [17].

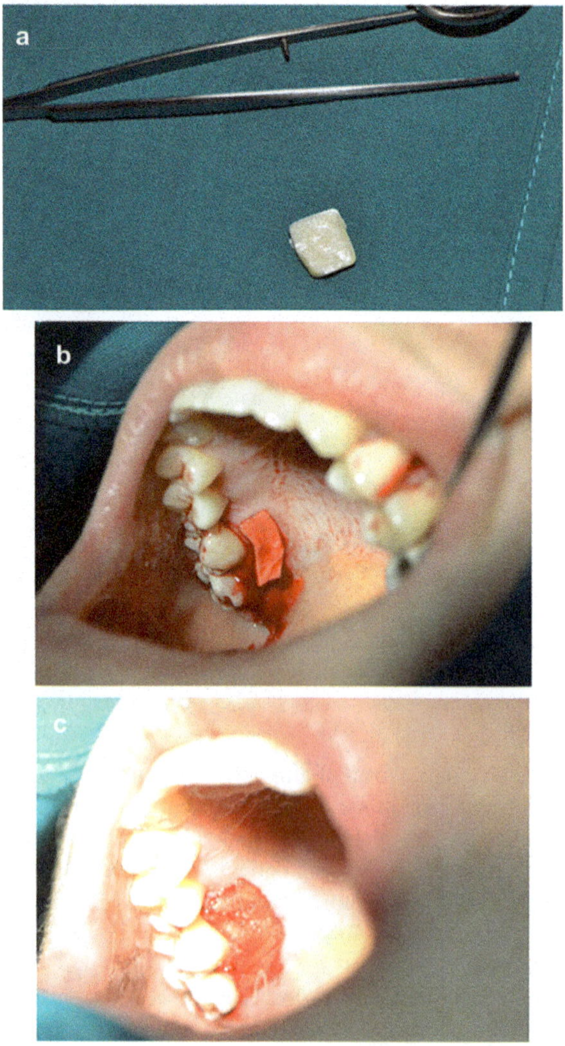

Fig. 27.5 (**a–c**) Use of chitosan to cover the palatal donor site following harvesting of a free mucosal autograft

Thrombin

Thrombin preparations (Thrombin-JMI®, Evithrom®, Thrombostat®, Thrombinar®, Thrombogen®, Recothrom®, and others) can be of animal origin (most commonly bovine) or human or recombinant. The use of human thrombin carries a theoretical risk of transmitting blood-borne viral infections (HIV, hepatitis B and C, and parvovirus B19) and prion infections (Creutzfeldt-Jakob disease). The use of bovine thrombin carries a risk of allergic reaction and a theoretical possibility of transmitting prion diseases. The mechanism of action of these agents is based on the direct conversion of fibrinogen into fibrin. Owing to its potent prothrombogenic effect, thrombin is used exclusively as a topical hemostatic agent. Thrombin preparations are most commonly available in powder form, which is mixed with physiological saline prior to use or applied directly to the wound. Thrombin can be used alone or in combination with other local hemostatic agents, such as gelatin, collagen, and ORC. The combination of thrombin and a gelatin matrix is most commonly used (Floseal®, Surgiflo®, and others). Thrombin is also one of the components of fibrin glue [3, 4, 6, 7, 13].

Fibrin Glue

Fibrin glue (Beriplast P®, Tissucol®, Evicel®, Quixil®, Tisseel®, TachoComb®, Crosseal®, and others) is a biological adhesive that mimics the final phase of the coagulation cascade at the surgical site, the conversion of fibrinogen into fibrin. It is a two-component system. One component consists of thrombin and calcium chloride, and the other of fibrinogen, coagulation factor XIII (FXIII), and an antifibrinolytic, most often aprotinin. In addition to commercial products, there is fibrin glue derived from a single donor's plasma, as well as autologous preparations obtained by cryoprecipitation from the patient's own blood. Fibrin glue is applied using a double-syringe system so that both components are mixed in equal amounts at the moment of application (Fig. 27.6a–d). The mechanism of action is as follows: in the presence of thrombin and calcium, fibrinogen is converted into fibrin, resulting in the formation of an unstable fibrin clot; FXIII stabilizes the clot, while an antifibrinolytic agent prevents its degradation (Fig. 27.7). Fibrin glue is considered one of the most effective hemostatic agents and can be used to control parenchymal and mild venous bleeding, secure sutures, and cover wounds. In addition to its adhesive and hemostatic properties, fibrin glue also accelerates wound healing and is completely biodegradable. Commercial products contain human-derived components. Therefore, despite rigorous donor selection and viral inactivation procedures that reduce the risk to a theoretical level, the possibility of transmitting blood-borne diseases cannot be entirely excluded. Such a risk does not exist in the case of autologous products, which are derived from the patient's own blood. One of the main disadvantages of these agents is their high cost [2, 6, 7, 13].

The effectiveness of fibrin glue as a local hemostatic agent has been proven after tooth extraction in patients on anticoagulant therapy [18], as well as in those with hemophilia and other congenital bleeding disorders [19–22].

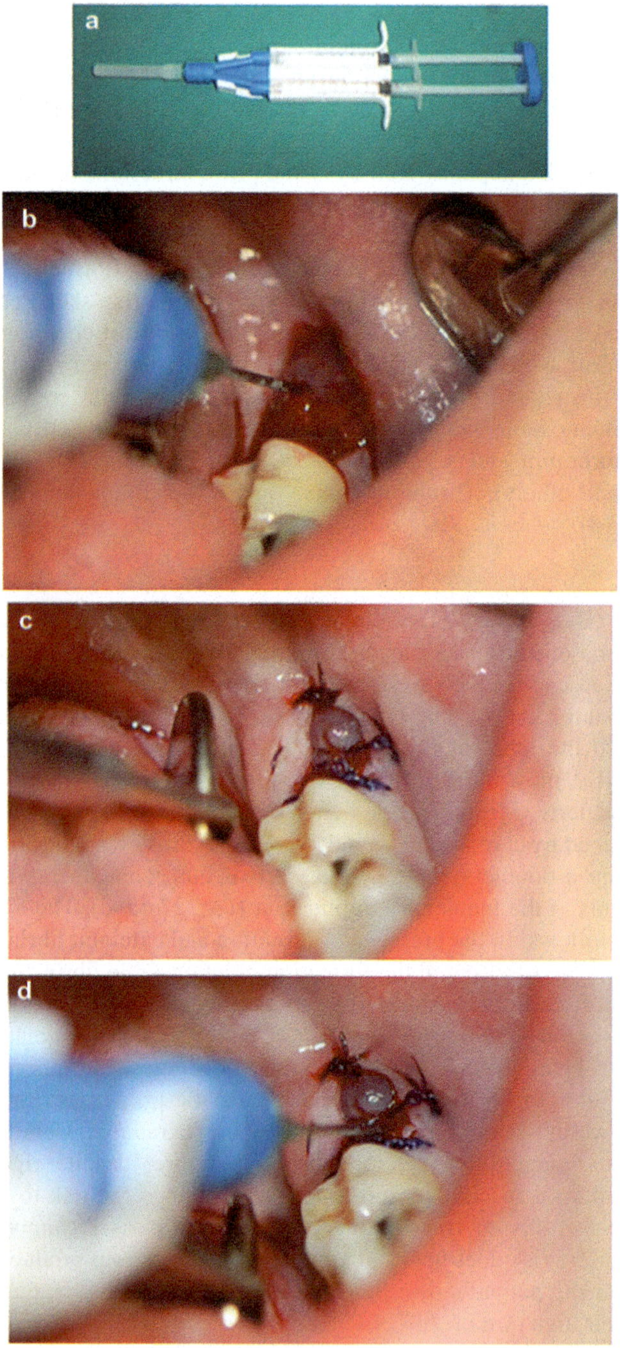

Fig. 27.6 (**a–d**) Application of fibrin glue following tooth extraction in a person with hemophilia

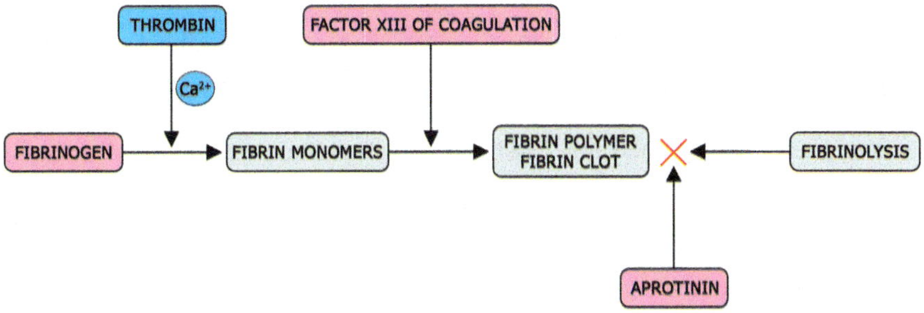

Fig. 27.7 Fibrin glue mechanism of action

Platelet-Rich Fibrin and Platelet-Rich Plasma

Platelet-rich fibrin (PRF) is an autologous preparation derived from the original platelet-rich plasma (PRP) formulation. Depending on the centrifugation process and preparation, the final product may vary, resulting in several forms of PRF, such as leukocyte platelet-rich fibrin (L-PRF), advanced platelet-rich fibrin (A-PRF), pure platelet-rich fibrin (P-PRF), injectable platelet-rich fibrin (I-PRF), and liquid platelet-rich fibrin (Liquid-PRF). These agents are primarily used in tissue regeneration and may accelerate wound healing. Although not classified as local hemostatic agents, some studies suggest that PRF and PRP preparations may be used to enhance local hemostasis following tooth extraction in patients taking anticoagulant therapy [23, 24] and in persons with hemophilia [25]. However, other studies indicate that these preparations are less effective than local hemostatic agents in preventing post-extraction bleeding in patients receiving oral anticoagulant therapy [17, 26].

Tissue Adhesives

Tissue adhesives are local hemostatic agents in the form of low-viscosity liquids that rapidly polymerize, forming a barrier that effectively seals the wound. They can be synthetic (cyanoacrylate glue, polyethylene glycol polymers) or semisynthetic (based on glutaraldehyde-albumin). They are primarily used to close skin wounds as an alternative to sutures. However, some of these agents can also be used within the oral cavity [27].

Cyanoacrylate glue (Histoacryl®, Omnex®, Dermabond®, and others) is composed of monomeric esters of cyanoacrylic acid. Its hemostatic effect is primarily achieved mechanically, owing to its ability to fill tissue defects and seal wounds due to exceptional adhesive properties. It also serves as a microbiological barrier. These agents require careful handling, as they strongly bind to various surfaces, including gloves, instruments, and surrounding tissues. The main reported adverse effect is the potential for an allergic reaction [1, 4, 6, 7].

There is limited data in the literature on the use of tissue adhesives for bleeding control after oral surgical procedures. Studies have reported the successful use of cyanoacrylate adhesive following tooth extraction in patients undergoing oral anticoagulant therapy [28].

Antifibrinolytics

Tranexamic acid (TA) (Capramol®, Lysteda®, and others), epsilon-aminocaproic acid (EACA) (Capramin®, Cyklokapron®, Amicar®, and others), and aprotinin are synthetic agents that prevent fibrinolysis of the coagulum by blocking the conversion of plasminogen to plasmin. Plasminogen and plasminogen activators are present in saliva and gingival crevicular fluid [29–31], and therefore the use of antifibrinolytics can be considered justified for preventing and treating bleeding following oral surgical procedures in patients with impaired hemostatic function. Aprotinin is one of the components of fibrin glue. Antifibrinolytic agents are available as tablets, granules, or ampoules for intravenous use.

Local use of antifibrinolytics has shown positive effects in the prevention of bleeding following oral surgical procedures in patients receiving vitamin K antagonist therapy [32–34], as well as in the management of mucosal bleeding or postoperative bleeding in the oral cavity in persons with hemophilia and other coagulopathies [35, 36]. Antifibrinolytics can be used systemically and locally.

In persons with hemophilia and other inherited coagulopathies, antifibrinolytics are used both systemically and locally, whereas in patients taking oral anticoagulant therapy, systemic administration is contraindicated because of the associated risk of thromboembolic events. Local application of these agents involves direct placement into the extraction socket, usually in combination with another local hemostatic, compression of the wound with a gauze soaked in an antifibrinolytic, or advising the patient to rinse the mouth with an antifibrinolytic solution.

TA is a synthetic derivative of the amino acid lysine. It achieves antifibrinolytic effect by reversible blockade of the lysine-binding sites on the plasminogen molecule. It is significantly more effective compared to EACA. When used as a mouthwash solution, the drug concentration in saliva remains sufficiently high for several hours after administration, while plasma levels are negligible, thereby avoiding undesirable systemic effects. A 4.8–5% TA solution is used as a mouth rinse in a volume of 10 ml. The solution is used for 2 min every 6 h, 2–7 days following tooth extraction [13, 35, 37].

Bone Wax

Bone wax (Bone Wax®, Waxocare®, Oriwax®, and others) is a mixture of beeswax, paraffin, and isopropyl palmitate. It is used to control minor bleeding from trabecular bone canaliculi. It is not indicated for use in cases of bleeding from a major blood vessel within the bone. Its mechanism of action is mechanical, providing a tamponade of the trabecular bone canals at the application site. It does not affect the physiological process of hemostasis. It is easily adapted and applied by pressing it onto the bleeding bony surface. The drawbacks of this agent include the inhibition of bone regeneration and osteogenesis, its non-biodegradable nature, and the potential to cause foreign body reactions, infection, and pain. Therefore, it is recommended that it be used in the minimum necessary amount, and any excess should be removed [3, 13]. It should not be used in sites where implant placement is planned, nor following bleeding from the mandibular canal due to the risk of paresthesia. There are also synthetic materials, such as alkylene oxide copolymer (e.g., Ostene®), which closely resembles bone wax in both its appearance and intended use. The material is easily applied to the bleeding surface, does not negatively affect osteogenesis, and is resorbed within 48 h [6, 37].

27.2 Local Hemostatic Measures

Local hemostatic methods include wound compression with gauze, ligation of the blood vessel, suturing of the wound, placement of a splint, and the use of heat for coagulation (thermocoagulation, electrocoagulation, and use of lasers).

To control or prevent bleeding following tooth extraction, the figure-of-eight suture technique is most commonly used (Fig. 27.8).

This suture technique stabilizes the blood clot, prevents displacement of the local hemostatic agent, and facilitates approximation of the wound edges after tooth extraction. Ligation of a blood vessel in the oral cavity is most commonly used to control bleeding following injury to the palatal blood vessels (Fig. 27.9). Bleeding following injury to the mandibular canal is most easily controlled by wound tamponade with iodoform gauze (Fig. 27.10). The gauze should be removed carefully several days after insertion to prevent disruption of the clot and recurrence of bleeding.

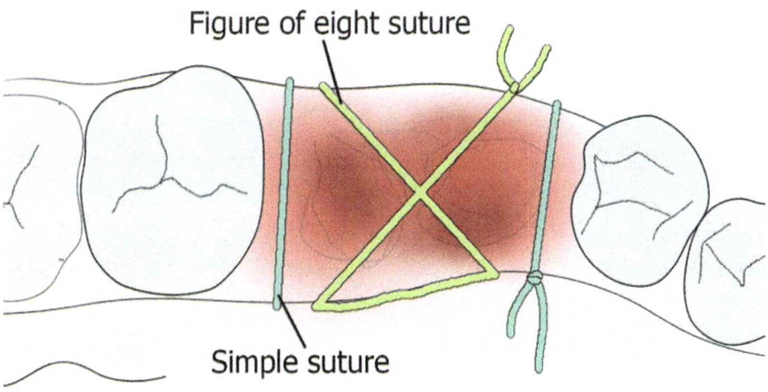

Fig. 27.8 Figure-of-eight suture technique

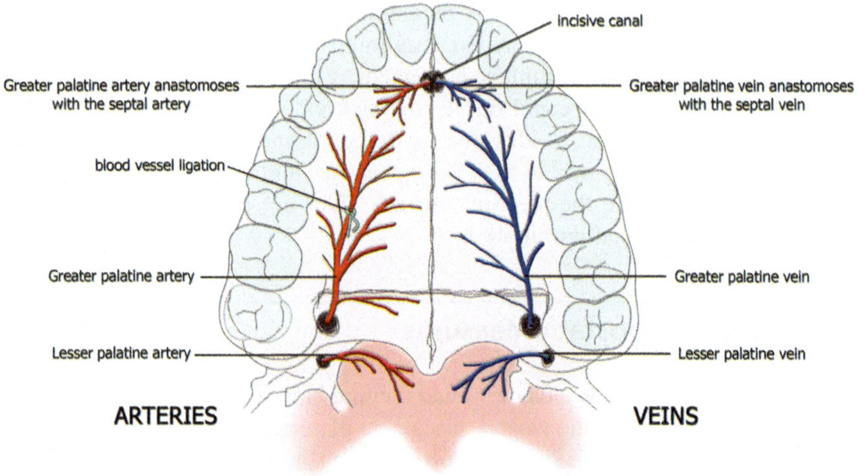

Fig. 27.9 Palatal blood vessels and their ligation

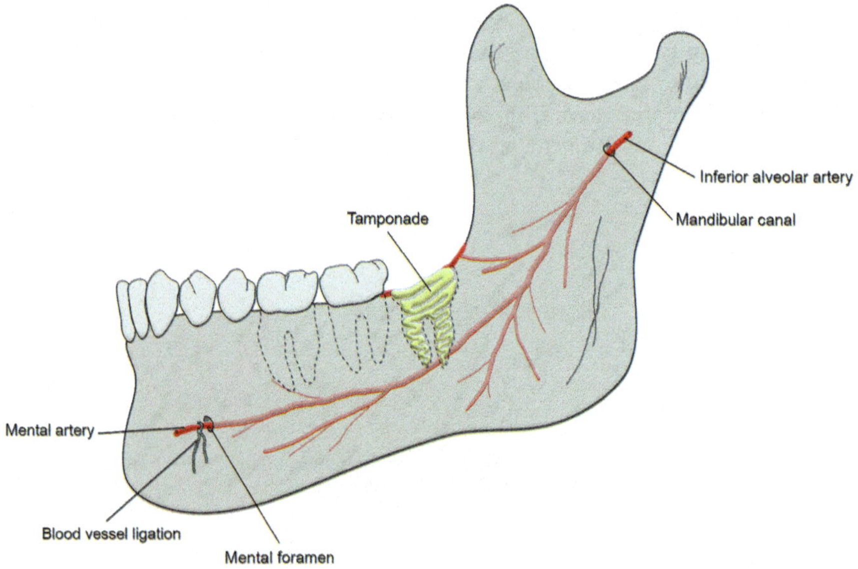

Fig. 27.10 Mandibular canal injury and iodoform gauze tamponade

Soft vacuum-formed splint is most commonly used after multiple tooth extractions in the same jaw in persons with hemophilia and other coagulopathies. Fabrication of a soft vacuum-formed splint begins with taking dental impressions before tooth extraction. After casting the model, the teeth scheduled for extraction are removed from the model, and the splint is fabricated to fully cover the extraction sites.

References

1. Belozerskaya GG, Makarov VA, Zhidkov EA, Malykhina LS, Sergeeva OA, Ter-Arutyunyants AA, et al. Local hemostatics (A review). Pharm Chem J. 2006;40:353–9.
2. Emilia M, Luca S, Francesca B, Luca B, Paolo S, Giuseppe F, Gianbattista B, Carmela M, Luigi M, Mauro L. Topical hemostatic agents in surgical practice. Transfus Apher Sci. 2011;45(3):305–11.
3. Lapierre F, D'Houtaud S, Wager M. Hemostatic agents in neurosurgery. In: Francesco Signorelli Explicative cases of controversial issues in neurosurgery. IntechOpen; 2012. p. 505–18.
4. Huang L, Liu GL, Kaye AD, Liu H. Advances in topical hemostatic agent therapies: a comprehensive update. Adv Ther. 2020;37(10):4132–48.
5. Spotnitz WD. Hemostats, sealants, and adhesives: a practical guide for the surgeon. Am Surg. 2012;78(12):1305–21.
6. Schonauer C, Mastantuoni C, Somma T, de Falco R, Cappabianca P, Tessitore E. Topical hemostatic agents in neurosurgery, a comprehensive review: 15 years update. Neurosurg Rev. 2022;45(2):1217–32.
7. Tompeck AJ, Gajdhar AUR, Dowling M, Johnson SB, Barie PS, Winchell RJ, King D, Scalea TM, Britt LD, Narayan M. A comprehensive review of topical hemostatic agents: the good, the bad, and the novel. J Trauma Acute Care Surg. 2020;88(1):e1–21.
8. Hilfenhaus J, Weidman E. Fibrin glue safety: inactivation of potential viral contaminants by pasteurization of the plasma components. Arzneimittelforschung. 1985;11:1617–9.
9. Mahardawi B, Jiaranuchart S, Rochanavibhata S, Arunjaroensuk S, Mattheos N, Pimkhaokham A. The role of hemostatic agents after tooth extractions: a systematic review and meta-analysis. J Am Dent Assoc. 2023;154(8):742–52.
10. Moreno-Drada JA, Abreu LG, Lino PA, Parreiras Martins MA, Pordeus IA, Guimarães N, de Abreu MH. Effectiveness of local hemostatic to prevent bleeding in dental patients on anticoagulation: a systematic review and network meta-analysis. J Craniomaxillofac Surg. 2021;49(7):570–83.
11. Nisi M, Carli E, Gennai S, Gulia F, Izzetti R. Hemostatic agents for the management of bleeding risk associated with oral anticoagulant therapy following tooth extraction: a systematic review. Appl Sci. 2022;12(21):11017.
12. Cziperle DJ. Avitene™ microfibrillar collagen hemostat for adjunctive hemostasis in surgical procedures: a systematic literature review. Med Devices (Auckl). 2021;14:155–63.
13. Scarano A, Leo L, Lorusso F, Tagariello G, Falisi G, Bugea C, Rapone B, Greco Lucchina A, Di Carmine MS. Topical hemostatic agents in oral surgery: a narrative review. Eur Rev Med Pharmacol Sci. 2023;27(3 Suppl):135–40.
14. Cakarer S, Eyupoglu E, Gunes CO, Kuseoglu BG, Berberoglu HK, Keskin. Evaluation of the hemostatic effects of Ankaferd blood stopper during dental extractions in patients on antithrombotic therapy. Clin Appl Thromb. 2013;19:96–9.
15. Kazancıoğlu HO, Cakır O, Ak G, Zülfikar B. The effectiveness of a new hemostatic agent (Ankaferd Blood Stopper) for the control of bleeding following tooth extraction in hemophilia: a controlled clinical trial. Turk J Haematol. 2013;30(1):19–24.
16. Lestari W, Yusry WNAW, Haris MS, Jaswir I, Idrus E. A glimpse on the function of chitosan as a dental hemostatic agent. Jpn Dent Sci Rev. 2020;56(1):147–54.
17. Katz MS, Ooms M, Heitzer M, Steiner T, Bock A, Peters F, Hölzle F, Modabber A. Platelet-rich fibrin as a hemostatic agent in dental extractions in patients taking anticoagulants or antiplatelet medication: a systematic review. Clin Oral Investig. 2024;28(11):587.
18. Bodner L, Weinstein JM, Baumgarten AK. Efficacy of fibrin sealant in patients on various levels of oral anticoagulant undergoing oral surgery. Oral Surg Oral Med Oral Pathol Oral Radiol Endod. 1998;86(4):421–4.
19. Bajkin BV, Rajic NV, Vujkov SB. Dental extraction in a hemophilia patient without factor replacement therapy: a case report. J Oral Maxillofac Surg. 2012;70(10):2276–7.
20. Kavakli E, Radomisli TE. Fibrin glue and clinical impact on haemophilia care. Haemophilia. 1999;5(6):392–6.

21. Suwannuraks M, Chuansumrit A, Sriudomporn N. The use of fibrin glue as an operative sealant in dental extraction in bleeding disorder patients. Haemophilia. 1999;5(2):106–8.
22. Correa ME, Annicchino-Bizzacchi JM, Jorge J Jr, Paes de Almeida O, Ozelo MC, Aranha FJ, et al. Clinical impact of oral health indexes in dental extraction of hemophilic patients. J Oral Maxillofac Surg. 2006;64(5):785–8.
23. Giudice A, Esposito M, Bennardo F, Brancaccio Y, Buti J, Fortunato L. Dental extractions for patients on oral antiplatelet: a within-person randomised controlled trial comparing haemostatic plugs, advanced-platelet-rich fibrin (A-PRF+) plugs, leukocyte- and platelet-rich fibrin (L-PRF) plugs and suturing alone. Int J Oral Implantol (Berl). 2019;12(1):77–87.
24. Brancaccio Y, Antonelli A, Barone S, Bennardo F, Fortunato L, Giudice A. Evaluation of local hemostatic efficacy after dental extractions in patients taking antiplatelet drugs: a randomized clinical trial. Clin Oral Investig. 2021;25(3):1159–67.
25. Cocero N, Pucci F, Messina M, Pollio B, Mozzati M, Bergamasco L. Autologous plasma rich in growth factors in the prevention of severe bleeding after teeth extractions in patients with bleeding disorders: a controlled comparison with fibrin glue. Blood Transfus. 2015;13:287–94.
26. Filho ELC, Franco JMPL, Ribeiro TR, Silva PGB, Costa FWG. Does platelet-rich fibrin prevent hemorrhagic complications after dental extractions in patients using oral anticoagulant therapy? J Oral Maxillofac Surg. 2021;79(11):2215–26.
27. Oladega AA, James O, Adeyemo WL. Cyanoacrylate tissue adhesive or silk suture for closure of surgical wound following removal of an impacted mandibular third molar: a randomized controlled study. J Craniomaxillofac Surg. 2019;47:93–8.
28. Al-Belasy FA, Amer MZ. Hemostatic effect of n-butyl-2- cyanoacrylate (histoacryl) glue in warfarin-treated patients undergoing oral surgery. J Oral Maxillofac Surg. 2003;61(12):1405–9.
29. Sindet-Pedersen S, Gram J, Jespersen J. Characterization of plasminogen activators in unstimulated and stimulated human whole saliva. J Dent Res. 1987;66:1199–203.
30. Gersel-Pedersen N. Fibrinolytic activity of blood and saliva before and after oral surgery. Int J Oral Surg. 1981;10(Suppl 1):114–21.
31. Majerus P, Dalcette B, Hermans M, Pourtois M, Capel P. Variations in fibrinolytic activity of human whole saliva. Eur J Oral Sci. 1996;104:341–5.
32. Carter G, Goss A. Tranexamic acid mouthwash-a prospective randomized study of a 2-day regimen vs 5-day regimen to prevent postoperative bleeding in anticoagulated patients requiring dental extractions. Int J Oral Maxillofac Surg. 2003;32(5):504–7.
33. Sindet-Pedersen S, Ramstrom G, Bernvil S, Blomback M. Hemostatic effect of tranexamic acid mouthwash in anticoagulant-treated patients undergoing oral surgery. N Engl J Med. 1989;320(13):840–3.
34. de Vasconcellos SJ, de Santana ST, Reinheimer DM, Faria-E-Silva AL, de Melo MF, Martins-Filho PR. Topical application of tranexamic acid in anticoagulated patients undergoing minor oral surgery: a systematic review and meta-analysis of randomized clinical trials. J Craniomaxillofac Surg. 2017;45(1):20–6.
35. Srivastava A, Santagostino E, Dougall A, Kitchen S, Sutherland M, Pipe SW, Carcao M, Mahlangu J, Ragni MV, Windyga J, Llinás A, Goddard NJ, Mohan R, Poonnoose PM, Feldman BM, Lewis SZ, van den Berg HM, Pierce GF, WFH Guidelines for the Management of Hemophilia panelists and co-authors. WFH guidelines for the management of hemophilia, 3rd edition. Haemophilia. 2020;Suppl 6:1–158. Erratum in: Haemophilia. 2021;27(4):699.
36. Bajkin B, Dougall A. Current state of play regarding dental extractions in patients with haemophilia: consensus or evidence-based practice? A review of the literature. Haemophilia. 2020;00:1–17.
37. Szumita RP, Szumita PM. Local techniques and pharmacological agents for management of bleeding in dentistry. In: Szumita RP, Szumita PM, editors. Hemostasis in dentistry. Cham: Springer; 2018. p. 187–99.

The manufacturer's authorised representative in the EU is Springer Nature Customer Service Centre GmbH, Europaplatz 3, 69115 Heidelberg, Germany. If you have any concerns regarding our products, please contact ProductSafety@springernature.com

Printed and bound by CPI Group (UK) Ltd, Croydon, CR0 4YY
05/10/2026
02228035-0001